Sticking To The
POINT

Sticking To The

Point

A Rational Methodology For The Step By Step Formulation & Administration Of A TCM Acupuncture Treatment

by
Bob Flaws

BLUE POPPY PRESS

Published by:

BLUE POPPY PRESS
1775 LINDEN AVE.
BOULDER, CO 80304

Second Edition, May, 1994

ISBN 0-936185-17-1

The information in this book is given in good faith. However, the translators and the publisher cannot be held responsible for any error or omission. Nor can they be held in any way responsible for treatment given on the basis of information contained in this book. The publisher make this information available to English language readers for scholarly and research purposes only.

The publishers do not advocate nor endorse self-medication by laypersons. Chinese medicine is a professional medicine. Laypersons interested in availing themselves of the treatments described in this book should seek out a qualified professional practitioner of Chinese medicine.

COMP Designation: Original work

Printed at Westview Press, Boulder, CO on acid free, recycled paper. ✪
Cover Printed at C&M Press, Thornton, CO.

10 9 8 7 6 5 4 3 2

Preface to Second Edition

Much has happened in the six years since I first wrote this book. However, as I continue to teach around the United States, the main problem I see in the teaching and learning of Traditional Chinese Medicine or TCM as a system has to do with language. As a profession, we have yet to adopt a standard technical terminology which is consistent and accurately reflects the Chinese literature from which our art derives.

This means that English-speaking practitioners are not using the same words with the same logic and implications as the Chinese doctors who created and continue to refine and expand this system. Not only is the language we are using frequently different in meaning and implication from our Chinese antecedents, but amongst Westerners, we may use any number of different English words to translate a single Chinese TCM technical term. Thus, English-speaking readers cannot cross-reference information in the English TCM literature with any degree of ease or confidence. It is difficult to know if the pulse image of one author is the same or different from the pulse image of another author. Some may call the *hua mai* a slippery pulse, a rolling pulse, a sliding pulse, or any number of alternatives. Yet in China, every TCM practitioner understands the same thing when they see *hua mai* in various books and periodicals.

Since publishing the first edition of this book, Nigel Wiseman and Ken Boss have brought out their *Glossary of Chinese Medical Terms and Acupuncture Points* published by Paradigm Publications. This book attempts to provide a standard list of translations of Chinese TCM technical terms. Although I continue

i

to find some of the translations Wiseman suggests awkward or hard to use, I basically accept his intent and methodology. As a teacher of TCM, I strongly believe our profession desperately needs a translationally accurate, standard technical vocabulary, and at the moment, even though it may not be perfect, Wiseman's glossary is the best we have.

Therefore, in editing this second edition, I have changed all the TCM technical terms to agree with Wiseman's terminology to the best of my ability. This will aid readers cross-reference the material in this book with other recent Blue Poppy Press releases, such as *Statements of Fact in TCM; How to Write a TCM Herbal Formula;* and *Sixty-seven Essential TCM Formulas for Beginners.* It will also help readers cross-reference the material contained herein with all of Paradigm Publications releases on TCM. And further, it allows readers to identify the Chinese characters implied by the English language words by looking these terms up in Wiseman's *Glossary.* Since English and Chinese are so dissimilar in their grammar and internal logic, no English translation can completely capture both the words, logic, and meaning of the Chinese, and, therefore, for those attempting to learn to read TCM in Chinese, knowing the original Chinese may provide even greater clarity and understanding.

In addition I have added several passages to more clearly explain what I was trying to say. I have also deleted several passages which were superfluous. Further, I have corrected a number of mistakes and reworded more than a few sentences. Hopefully, these changes will allow this book to be of use to Western practitioners for another few years.

Bob Flaws, April, 1994

Table of Contents

Preface to the Second Edition i

1   Introduction 1

2   Diagnosis 5

3   Therapeutic Principles 21

4   Choosing Points Based on Principle (1) 45

5   Choosing Points Based on Principle (2) 99

6   Composing the Acupuncture Formula 109

7   Acupuncture Administration 119

8   Conclusion 137

Bibliography 139

Index 141

1

Introduction

T ravelling around the country giving graduate level seminars to American acupuncturists and practitioners of Traditional Chinese Medicine or TCM, I have become acutely aware of the general lack of clarity in American practitioners concerning the methodology of our profession. For me, one of the greatest values of TCM is its time-tested methodology. To a large extent, this methodology is based on the logic inherent in the Chinese language. In Chinese, TCM is extremely clear and logical. However, in translation, this logic and clarity are often lost. Frequently, the immediately perceived connections between two Chinese words to a Chinese reader do not carry over to the two (or more) English words chosen to translate them. Nigel Wiseman, Andrew Ellis, and Ken Boss, also aware of this problem, have attempted to rectify it by creating a standard English vocabulary which hews as closely as possible to the Chinese in their *Fundamentals of Chinese Medicine.*[1] Although many may feel uncomfortable, as I myself do, with some of their neologisms, I believe their endeavor correctly addresses the main problem with the teaching and practice of TCM in the English-speaking today.

The process of doing TCM is based on a relatively rigorous methodology and logic. This system of logic is like calculus or a

---

1 *Fundamentals of Chinese Medicine*, compiled, translated, and amended by Andrew Ellis, Nigel Wiseman, and Ken Boss, Paradigm Publications, Brookline, MA, 1985

computer language. Only if one uses the correct terms in their proper sequence will one get the proper, time-tested, clinically verified result at the end. Doing TCM in English is often like adding apples and oranges. Because of misunderstanding the denotations and connotations of the technical Chinese TCM terminology, we Western practitioners all too often plug into our clinical equations the wrong information or else process the right information with the wrong system of logic.

For instance, equating the *wei qi* with the immune system is an oft repeated misconception that has led a number of Western practitioners to offer categorically mistaken treatments to numerous patients. *Wei qi* as a technical concept in TCM has a very specific definition. 1) It warms the body, both the exterior and the interior. 2) It defends the exterior from penetration specifically by the *liu yin* or six environmental excesses. 3) It opens and closes the pores. And 4) it circulates primarily outside the twelve regular channels (*shi er zheng jing*) and circulates according to a diurnal rhythm. During the day it circulates in the exterior and at night it retreats to the interior. It is produced from the pure of the impure in the lower burner but it is commanded or governed by the lungs. As such, the *wei qi* is not identical to any single concept in modern Western medicine.

Likewise the TCM concept *gan* or liver is not identical to the Western biological liver. According to the TCM definition of *gan*, the liver controls coursing and discharge and stores the blood. *And it is located on the left!* The Chinese liver categorically does not purify the blood and, in fact, in TCM, there is no concept of blood purification as such. We may talk about clearing the blood, but that specifically means clearing heat from the *xue fen* or blood division.

At the Dechen Yonten Dzo Institute of Buddhist Medicine (no longer existent), we attempted to address this issue by requiring all our students to learn to read medical Chinese from a medically trained, native speaker. It is my experience that the closer one follows the time-tested methodology of Chinese medicine as formulated in Chinese, the better the clinical results. However, the majority of American practitioners, it seems, neither have the time nor inclination to learn Chinese. Therefore, I am offering this small book on the methodology for the step by step formulation and administration of an acupuncture treatment in an attempt to clarify the practice of TCM in the West.

The material in this book is based on lectures given by me at Dechen Yonten Dzo.[2] It also includes various translations from Chinese sources done by our faculty and students and lecture notes from Dr. (Eric) Tao Xi-yu and Dr. Xi Yang-jiang. Transcription, collation, research, and editing were done by Honora Lee Wolfe, Nina Steinway, Rose Crescenz, and Dennis Brooks.

Although I have stated elsewhere that the creation of acupuncture formulas mimicking the creation of Chinese herbal formulas does not most clearly express the fact that what acupuncture pre-eminently and inherently does is to balance the flow of qi and blood, based on my experience trying to teach TCM in the United States, I have come to the conclusion that this methodology does provide the relative beginner with an exceptionally clear, step by step protocol. As such, it provides a firm foundation upon which the practitioner can build and from which one can branch out as their knowledge and experience become more sophisticated.

Among a certain segment of the population most interested in Chinese medicine in the West, intuition is valued above rationality. However, for me, intuition is merely the clarity of

---

[2] The Dechen Yonten Dzo offered a two-year acupuncture training in Boulder, CO from 1985 to 1989.

knowing something so well that one does not need to consciously and deliberately move through all the propositions of a syllogism. For me, the difference between rationality and intuition is merely speed and, in my experience, training oneself to think clearly and logically is the quickest and surest path to insight. In addition, if one merely relies on intuition, sometimes one will be right and sometimes one will be wrong. If one thinks through a problem step by step in a rational manner, this margin for error diminishes and, even when one is wide of the mark, it will usually not be by much. Since the first rule of therapeutics is to first do no harm, such a rational process helps diminish the possibility of causing the patient even further suffering or detriment to their life.

The practice of medicine is not a business, or at least it should not be. It is a sacred trust. Each patient comes to us entrusting us with their health and life itself. By taking the time and care to step by step think through their diagnosis and treatment, we honor their trust and act in an appropriately responsible and professional way. The logic of TCM has been carefully honed by two millennia of professional practitioners who, for the most part, acknowledged and accepted the sacred trust inherent in their calling. It is my hope that this small book will help establish and continue this exceptionally clear methodology here in the West.

In brief, this methodology can be summed up as the logical progression from diagnosis to therapeutic principles to treatment plan and from thence to treatment application. Although this book is about the creation of specifically TCM acupuncture treatments, this same methodology can be applied to the erection of TCM-style herbal medicine, dietary therapy, massage therapy, and even exercise plans.

2

Diagnosis

A good TCM pattern diagnosis is the essential prerequisite of a good TCM acupuncture treatment. Although this is axiomatic in that one must first understand what is wrong before one can attempt to fix it, diagnosis is the most difficult aspect of TCM to master. One's ability as a practitioner of TCM is largely a function of how good a diagnostician one is. Relatively reliable information on the four examinations *(si zhen)* is currently available in English, as are expositions on the eight (guiding) principles *(ba gang)*, and the main patterns (of disharmony) or *zheng*. Sources of well translated, basic factual information on these topics are listed in the bibliography.

However, after memorizing the lists of signs and symptoms correlating to the eight principles, the tongue, the pulse, and the major *zheng*, all too often, Western practitioners are not clear about how to analyze, synthesize, and utilize these voluminous bits of information. *One of the most important realizations for Western practitioners of TCM is that Chinese medicine only treats logically and methodologically "Chinese" diseases.*[3]

---

[3] This is a bit of an over-simplification. In the last 15 years, Chinese TCM practitioners have created TCM pattern discrimination breakdowns for modern Western disease categories.

Disease Diagnosis

English language texts on Chinese medicine which, when discussing pathology, begin with modern Western medical disease categories tend to obscure the logic inherent in the Chinese categorization of disease. A very clear example of such translational obfuscation is David Owen's translation of *tan yin* (phlegm rheum) as gastritis in Felix Mann's *The Treatment Of Disease By Acupuncture.*[4] Under the Chinese heading *tan yin,* there are four subdivisions which, as constellations of signs and symptoms, have little or nothing to do with gastritis.[5] Therefore, a Western practitioner with a patient whose major complaint is gastritis may be perplexed that their patient does not conform to any of the *zheng* or patterns listed.

In other words, the Chinese map of disease categorizes the human experience of disease differently than modern Western medicine. It draws different boundaries around different sets of signs and symptoms based on its different theories of disease causation and evolution and on its different methods of diagnosis. However, saying that TCM only logically treats Chinese categories of disease does not mean that TCM only treats Chinese people in China. It is my experience that the TCM map of disease by and large does cover adequately and universally the terrain of human disease.

For instance, a Western practitioner may be perplexed that vaginitis and vaginal lesions, such as herpes genitalia, are not a

---

[4] Mann, Felix, *The Treatment of Disease by Acupuncture*, William Heinemann Medical Books, Ltd, London, 1980, p. 95

[5] These four subdivisions are phlegm rheum, suspended rheum, overflowing rheum, and branch rheum.

category of disease in standard Chinese *fu ke* or gynecology texts.[6] That is because *fu ke* is a subdivision of *nei ke* or internal medicine. Vaginal lesions, occurring on the outside of the body or *wai*, are categorized as a *wai ke* or external medicine problem and are described in detail in *wai ke* texts.[7] Similarly, PID is also not found in traditional Chinese *fu ke* texts. Yet TCM treats women whose Western medical diagnosis is PID extremely well. In such cases, the Traditional Chinese categories of disease are most often *shao fu tong* (lower abdominal pain) and *dai xia* (abnormal vaginal discharge). Within these general Chinese disease categories, detailed, logical subdivisions are discriminated in the Chinese literature.

Since Western patients seeking Chinese medical treatment typically express their major complaint in terms of a previously established or subjectively assumed modern Western medical diagnosis, the first step in establishing a TCM diagnosis is to identify the general Chinese category of disease. By disease category I do not mean pattern, such as liver depression, qi stagnation or kidney/spleen yang vacuity. By Chinese disease category, I mean those headings found in traditional Chinese treatment manuals,[8] such as *shang han* (cold damage), *wen bing* (warm disease), *wu lin* (the five stranguries), *qi shan* (the seven *shan* conditions pertaining to the

---

[6] For instance, Song Guang-ji and Yu Xiao-zhen's *A Handbook of Traditional Chinese Gynecology*, translated by Zhang Ting-liang, Blue Poppy Press, Boulder, CO, 1987.

[7] Dermatology, or *pi fu ke* is a part of *wai ke*, and a section on vaginal lesions appears in Liang Jian-hui's, *A Handbook of Traditional Chinese Dermatology*, translated by Zhang Ting-liang and Bob Flaws, Blue Poppy Press, Boulder, CO, 1988, p. 45-46.

[8] For instance, Xiao Shao-qing's *Zhong Guo Zhen Jiu Chu Fang Xue (The Theory of Writing Prescriptions in Chinese Acupuncture*, Ning Xia, PRC, 1986

groin and genitalia), *yue jing xian qi* (menstruation ahead of schedule), *tong jing* (painful menstruation), etc. With a knowledge of such Chinese disease categories, one can then find detailed discussions and differential discriminations of these diseases in the Chinese TCM literature.

Pattern Discrimination

However, even without access to the Chinese literature, once one has identified the general Chinese category of disease, one can usually logically deduce the *zheng* or pattern (of disharmony) from a basic application of the four examinations, the eight principles, and pattern discrimination *(bian zheng)*. In fact, that is the beauty of Chinese medicine. If one knows how to apply the four examinations and how to discriminate patterns, one can logically diagnose and methodologically treat diseases even without prior knowledge of the disease entity. This is because TCM as a particular style of Chinese medicine bases its treatment more on pattern discrimination than on disease diagnosis. Thus it is said in Chinese,

Yi bing tong zhi,
Tong bing yi zhi.

One disease, different treatments,
Different diseases, one treatment.

This means that two patients with the same disease may receive two very different treatments at the hands of a TCM practitioner. This is because, although their disease diagnosis is the same, their patterns are different. Likewise, two patients diagnosed with different diseases may receive essentially the same treatment because their patterns are the same. This basing of treatment on pattern discrimination *(bian zheng lun zhi)* is the defining

8

characteristic of TCM as a particular style of Chinese medicine. Although every patient with the same disease must have certain defining or pathognomonic signs and symptoms, they may also have a number of other signs and symptoms which vary from patient to patient. It is the entirety of a patient's signs and symptoms which define a TCM *zheng* or pattern, and in TCM, the entire pattern is given preeminence in guiding treatment over the particular disease. This is because the disease is merely a figure within the ground of the pattern, while the pattern describes the entirety of the patient's condition.

In TCM, there are 10 broad categories of *bian zheng* or pattern discrimination. These are:

1. Five phase pattern discrimination (*wu xing bian zheng*)
2. Eight principle pattern discrimination (*ba gang bian zheng*)
3. Qi and blood pattern discrimination (*qi xue bian zheng*)
4. Fluids and humors pattern discrimination (*jin ye bian zheng*)
5. Viscera and bowels pattern discrimination (*zang fu bian zheng*)
6. Channel and connecting vessel pattern discrimination (*jing luo bian zheng*)
7. Disease cause pattern discrimination (*bing yin bian zheng*)
8. Six division pattern discrimination (*liu fen bian zheng*)
9. Defensive, qi, constructive, and blood pattern discrimination (*wei qi ying xue bian zheng*)
10. Three burners pattern discrimination (*san jiao bian zheng*)

Although there are these ten broad categories of patterns that can be discriminated in TCM, in clinical practice, typically the pattern that gets written on the patient's chart is made up of elements of several of these types of patterns. For instance, in a wind cold external invasion pattern, this pattern is made up of disease cause (*bing yin*) and eight principle (*ba gang*) discriminations. Wind identifies the disease cause, while cold and the fact that the disease is in the exterior are two of the eight principles. Or, if one writes down that their patient is manifesting a liver blood vacuity pattern, this is made up of elements of eight principle, qi and blood (*qi xue*), and viscera and bowel (*zang fu*) pattern discriminations. The fact that the pattern is identified with the liver is a viscera and bowel discrimination. The fact that the pattern is identified with the blood is a qi and blood discrimination, and the fact that the pattern is identified as vacuity is an eight principle discrimination. In the same way, most of the patterns patients exhibit are made up of elements of more than one of these 10 types of discrimination.

TCM patterns are, by their very nature, more general and broad than diseases. For instance, if a patient complains of a skin lesion, it is relatively unimportant whether this is, from a modern Western medical point of view, eczema, psoriasis, or neurodermatitis, or even, from a Chinese point of view, *shi zheng, ying xie bing,* or *shen jing xing pi yan*, which in fact are only the Chinese translations of the previous Western medical terms. What is important is the practitioner's ability to analyze the lesions according to the logic of TCM. Redness and inflammation are manifestations of heat. Itching is a manifestation of wind. Suppuration is a manifestation of dampness. Purulence is a manifestation of toxins. And scaling is a manifestation of dryness and insufficiency of blood and fluids. In the case of skin lesions of all sorts, the practitioner parses out the nature of the lesion depending upon the relative proportions of these qualities of the lesion. If a skin lesion is red, itchy, and scaly, it exhibits the pattern of heat, wind, and dryness. The practitioner next tabulates the patient's other systemic signs and symptoms and their tongue and pulse. These, likewise, should also be manifestations of heat and insufficiency of blood and fluids. For instance, we might expect a dry, slightly crevassed, red tongue and a fine, fast pulse.

Next, he or she must posit a disease mechanism or dynamic (*bing ji)* which, according to the theories of TCM, would account for such lesions in the particular patient at hand. In the above example, these lesions and accompanying signs and symptoms may be due to heat in the liver being transferred to the blood with a concomitant drying out of the blood giving rise to stirring of internal wind in the exterior. Questioning the patient as to diet, lifestyle, and the history of their condition and related symptoms would then confirm or deny this hypothesis. In other words, one should check for the presence or absence of causative factors which might cause heat in the liver, such as stress, emotional upset, alcohol, and/or a preponderance of greasy, spicy foods in the diet.

If one does have access to a good differential breakdown of disease entities, one begins by discriminating between the patterns listed for the particular Chinese disease. For instance, if a patient presents with muscular flaccidity, numbness, loss of strength, and loss of voluntary movement, the traditional Chinese disease category is *wei zheng* or atony pattern. According to Dr. Ou-yang Yi, the *zheng* or patterns (of disharmony) most commonly accounting for *wei zheng* are: 1) insufficiency of lung yin, 2) detriment and damage of the liver and kidneys, 3) spleen vacuity with insufficiency of transportation, 4) retention of damp heat, 5) blood stasis in the channels and connecting vessels, 6) phlegm congelation and hidden evil fluid, and 7) flowing discharge of phlegm rheum. Detriment and damage of the liver and kidneys is further subdivided into: a) malnutrition of the sinews and bones due to insufficiency of liver blood and kidney essence; b) prenatal insufficiency, remembering that the blood and essence share a common source, *i.e.*, the kidneys, the prenatal viscus; and c) inability of yang to warm the channels and moisten the sinews because of failure in propelling the blood and fluids. Spleen vacuity is further subdivided into: a) malnutrition of the flesh and muscles due to the spleen not transforming the *ying* and blood and

b) malfunction in the qi dynamic *vis à vis* transportation of fluids.[9] Interestingly, phlegm stasis and hidden evil fluid and flowing discharge of phlegm rheum are two of the subdivisions of *tan yin* above mistranslated as supposed varieties of the Western medical disease gastritis.

Individually Tailoring the Pattern Discrimination

At first glance, such a detailed discrimination of the different types of *wei zheng* make it seem that all the practitioner needs to do is match their patient's signs and symptoms with the signs and symptoms of one of these *zheng*, and, in theory, that is correct. However, in practice, often one finds that their patient's condition is not adequately and solely described by one or another of the listed patterns. Such textbook patterns describe hypothetical pure types and they are presented this way for didactic reasons. They are simplifications idealized in order to maximally contrast with the other patterns listed. But, in clinical practice, one rarely encounters such simple cases and pure types. Each pattern listed implies a different disease dynamic, but it is not uncommon for a patient's condition to be caused by two different, although often indirectly related mechanisms. In such cases, the patient's signs and symptoms will be a mixture of certain of the signs and symptoms of more than one pattern. They will not fall into such neat, discreet groupings. In such cases, the practitioner must take care to analyze each sign and symptom both individually and as a whole.

Even in the face of a welter of confusing and seemingly contradictory signs and symptoms, one starts by parsing each out,

---

[9] Ou-yang Yi, *Handbook of Differential Diagnosis & Treatment*, Vol. 3, trans. by C. S. Cheung, Harmonious Sunshine Cultural Center, San Francisco, 1987, p. 61-65

beginning from what is known and hypothesizing about what is only surmised until the complete, detailed, and individualized description of the patient's pattern (of disharmony) emerges. Such individualized pattern diagnoses depend upon a sound knowledge of TCM theories of *bing ji* or disease dynamics and a faith in playing what one sees as opposed to what one expects. It is of utmost importance that the final diagnosis be tailored to fit the patient and not the patient be made to fit the diagnosis by conveniently discounting certain seeming anomalies.

Different TCM textbooks often give somewhat different breakdowns for the same disease. For instance, *Essentials of Chinese Acupuncture* only lists lung heat, damp heat, and insufficiency of the liver and kidney essence as *zheng* accounting for *wei* or atony.[10] In the absence of a fuller exposition such as Dr. Ou-yang Yi's above, it is imperative to simply tally up the various signs and symptoms and to see what they add up to. Even if they do not correspond to a listed *zheng* for the disease at hand in the currently available literature, if one can account according to the TCM theories of disease dynamics for how such an imbalance could cause *wei zheng,* one should proceed from that diagnosis.

Case History

The following case history exemplifies how one individualizes a complicated diagnosis based on an understanding of the individual signs and symptoms in the light of TCM theories of disease dynamics.

---

[10] *Essentials of Chinese Acupuncture*, ed. by Cheng Xin-nong, Foreign Language Press, Beijing, 1980, p. 371

The patient was a 39 year old woman with a confirmed modern Western medical diagnosis of MS. She had been diagnosed several years previously and was presently confined to a wheelchair. Both her left arm and leg were partially paralyzed. Her foot was occasionally spastic. She did not experience numbness. She was overweight, had facial acne, and tended to be constipated with hard, compacted stools. She was heat sensitive but did *not* sweat. There was some urinary incontinence and she had recently had problems with dysuria and urgency. In addition, for some time she had suffered from a shortened menstrual cycle (21 days) *and* menorrhagia. Her tongue was a little pale and extremely fluted. The coating was light yellow on the rear two thirds but geographic to the front with a bald patch behind the tip and to the left side with a red tip and a red rim around this patch. Her pulse was deep, very fine, weak, and fast.

Analysis of Signs & Symptoms

Analyzing this patient's signs and symptoms, tongue, and pulse, the TCM pattern discrimination is lung heat (vacuity) above, heat in the stomach but vacuity and dampness of the spleen in the middle, and damp heat below. In addition, there was internal stirring of wind due to insufficiency of blood in turn due to the spleen not transforming the blood and excessive menstrual bleeding. This meno-metrorrhagia was due to both the liver not storing the blood because of heat and deficient qi not restraining the blood. In fact, this patient had some elements of four of the ten *zheng* listed by Dr. Ou-yang above and her *wei zheng* was not simply due to one or the other.

Her lack of sweat, intolerance to heat, occasional urinary incontinence, and acne plus the geographic tongue tip and fast, fine pulse all suggest vacuity heat in the lungs. Her yellow tongue fur and hard compacted stools and again her acne suggest stomach heat most probably due to long-term accumulation of stagnant food. Her obesity and scalloped tongue plus weak and deep pulse suggest spleen qi vacuity probably due to long-term retention of dampness. The damp heat is suggested by the yellowish coating to the rear of the tongue, the history of dysuria and urgency, and the theoretical tendency of dampness to percolate downward, *i.e.* to the lower burner. Insufficiency of blood giving rise to internal stirring of wind is evidenced by the pale tongue, fine pulse, tendency to hard, compacted stools, history of excessive and too frequent menstrual bleeding, and muscular spasticity. In general, this excessive menstrual bleeding was probably due to a combination of *both* long-standing heat and qi vacuity — the heat causing the blood to flow recklessly outside its pathways and the (spleen) qi failing to hold or restrain the blood within its vessels.

Such a complex diagnosis and detailed, point for point analysis of the patient's signs and symptoms are what is required when dealing with the majority of Western patients who, for a variety of reasons, do not conform to the simple *zheng* listed in textbooks. Such textbook *zheng* are merely the building blocks of a final diagnosis. Most patients' problems are not so discreet. Additionally, the beginner is cautioned not to immediately assign a meaning to any given sign or symptom until seen in relation to the entire constellation. The final meaning or cause of any sign or symptom ultimately depends upon an understanding of the *bing ji* or disease dynamic and not on just the rote memorization of lists of correspondences.

Writing the Pattern Discrimination in the Patient's Chart

It is quite important that the practitioner not only formulate such a precise and detailed, individual pattern diagnosis but that they write this down on the patient's chart. All too often, Western practitioners will begin the discussion of case histories with a

15

modern Western diagnosis and a review of the treatments they gave and not the patient's TCM pattern discrimination. This is a great mistake since *only proceeding from a rationally arrived at TCM pattern discrimination can one derive a rational TCM acupuncture treatment plan.* And, when writing such a diagnosis down, the practitioner must take care to note this diagnosis in the agreed upon, standard professional terms. The diagnostic parameters of these terms are standardized and the practitioner should try to be as precise and accurate as possible. There are definite, specific signs and symptoms which differentiate liver depression, qi stagnation from depressive heat. These two different diagnoses require different treatment. These TCM patterns and their parameters are, for the most part, available in already existing English language texts.

Having a vague notion that something is wrong with a patient's liver is not enough. Qin Bo-wei, in his essay, "*Gan Bing (Liver Disease)*", lists 20 ways that Chinese TCM practitioners agree the TCM liver may become imbalanced.[11] Having written down the patient's key signs and symptoms, tongue, and pulse and the pattern discrimination based on these, other professional practitioners are then able to assess whether, in fact, this pattern discrimination is correct or incorrect. Then, sharing such case histories, we all can learn from our mistakes and advance in our art. For instance, if one writes down that a patient is suffering from liver fire but cannot substantiate the presence of pathogenic heat by any sign or symptom, this is then an erroneous diagnosis and treatment based on such an erroneous diagnosis will likely to be erroneous as well. In other words, a professional TCM pattern

---

[11] Qin Bo-wei, "Gan Bing (Liver Disease)", *Qin Bo-wei's Medical Essays*, Hunan Science and Technology Press, 1981, p. 285-334. An English language version of a number of essays from this book has been translated by Charles Chace and will be published by Paradigm Publications in 1994 or 1995.

discrimination should be objectively grounded in a rational analysis of signs and symptoms according to agreed upon professional norms.

When analyzing signs and symptoms the practitioner must understand not just that a sign usually means this or that but the mechanics of how a sign is produced. This means the practitioner needs to understand the logic behind the causation of various signs and symptoms. If the pulse is fine one needs to understand that the *size* of the pulse when smaller than normal primarily relates to substance. Therefore, a fine pulse indicates less than normal substance. In TCM, substance *vis à vis* the pulse means blood, yin, or fluids and humors. Understanding that, then one determines which of these is insufficient based on other corroborating signs and symptoms. Whereas, strength is an indication of function and function *vis à vis* the pulse means qi.

Or, take for example speed. The speed of the pulse traditionally tells us about heat in the organism, both righteous and evil. But, if we think deeper about the speed of the pulse, it is a function again of the qi, since the qi moves the blood, and heat is nothing other than qi, since qi is, by nature, warm. If the pulse is fast and skips beats, then this is the qi moving so rapidly that it is coming apart from the blood every so often. When the practitioner can go a little deeper like this in understanding the mechanics of causation, then one does not have to depend upon memorization or reference books, but can figure things out for themselves.

The Four Examinations & Western Medicine

Also, the signs and symptoms which can be used to logically deduce a TCM pattern diagnosis are only those that can be collected by the traditional four examinations. All information concerning the patient's disease which a traditional Chinese doctor could not know by either observing, hearing/smelling, palpating, or questioning are not germane to the process of making a TCM pattern diagnosis. For instance, it is my opinion that lab test reports should almost never be fudged into the equation of making a TCM pattern diagnosis. Such extraneous information tends to distort the logic of the self-contained TCM process. Such information may help the practitioner assess the gravity of the case or may help them decide if Chinese medicine should be resorted to in the present case, but such information should not be used to make the TCM pattern discrimination itself.

A patient may come with a lab report confirming, from a modern Western medical point of view, that they have nephritis. But, from the four examinations, all the TCM practitioner knows is that the patient has superficial edema which comes and goes and has been occurring for a long time. At this point, the TCM practitioner should also know that the patient's traditional Chinese disease diagnosis is *shui zhong*, water swelling or edema. This edema is worse in their four extremities and is also characterized as pitting. Their body feels very heavy and they are fatigued. Their digestion is sluggish and their upper abdomen is distended. They also have a yellow, puffy facial complexion. Their tongue is fat with teeth marks on its border, and their pulse is soft (*ruan*) and relaxed/retarded (*huan*).

According to the logic of TCM, these signs and symptoms add up to the TCM pattern of spleen dampness. In this case, the lab findings confirming nephritis might lead the practitioner astray and to treat the *wrong* Chinese viscus if they were used to establish the TCM pattern diagnosis. This goes back once again to the necessity of understanding that TCM is a self-contained conceptual system and of being clear about the internal logic and parameters of this system. The defining parameters of TCM *zheng* are *only* the signs and symptoms, tongue, and pulse gathered by the four examinations.[12] However, knowing that the patient has nephritis, the modern TCM practitioner does know something about the severity and prognosis of this patient's condition that the TCM pattern alone does not necessarily reveal.

Diseases & Patterns

Western patients and practitioners alike will often ask, however, "Doesn't the patient *really* have nephritis?" Yes, on a material, modern Western medical level, they do. That may be their modern Western medical *disease* diagnosis. But they just as really exhibit the pattern of spleen dampness. These two seemingly contradictory diagnoses are two different maps or conceptualizations of reality and in no way negate or invalidate each other. The modern Western disease exists within the ground of the patient's total pattern. Therefore, the TCM pattern should include and subsume the disease diagnosis, not contradict it. However, when it comes to treatment, TCM protocols are logically correlated to TCM patterns (of disharmony). Further, TCM practitioners emphasize the basing of their treatment on the pattern as opposed to the disease. In addition and, from the patient's point of view, more importantly, TCM treatment given on the basis of such traditional pattern discrimination is effective in our world and in our patients. For our patients, that is the bottom line. Treating kidney channel

---

[12] In the People's Republic of China, research is underway to correlate various lab reports and microscopic findings with TCM *zheng* or patterns. For instance, RBCs, WBCs, microcirculation under the nails, and serum antibodies or hormone levels have all been tested to see if, in a particular disease, particular anomalies are correlated with particular patterns. Although in certain cases there is a statistical preponderance of certain lab findings with certain patterns in certain diseases, these are not absolute. In other words, 75% of persons with a particular disease having a certain blood analysis may exhibit a yin vacuity pattern, but that still leaves 25% of patients with the same blood work who exhibit a different pattern.

points or administering Chinese kidney medicinals when the patient's TCM pattern diagnosis is spleen dampness, categorically, will not make the patient better and might conceivably make them worse. This point cannot be stressed too often or too strongly.

3

Therapeutic Principles

I n Chinese TCM clinics, the next step in ultimately treating the
patient is to logically deduce and state on the patient's chart the
therapeutic principles necessary to rebalance or rectify the
imbalance implied by the pattern diagnosis. The basic therapeutic
philosophy of Chinese medicine is heteropathy. This means that
the doctor supplies or recommends the introduction of the equal
opposite qi in order to restore balance within the organism. This
doctrine of heteropathy is based on Chapter 74 of the *Nei Jing Su
Wen (Internal Classic, Simple Questions)*:

> In treating various kinds of victorious and revengeful energies, a
> cold disease should be heated, a hot disease should be made cold,
> a warm disease should be cooled, and a cool disease should be
> warmed, a dispersing disease should secured, and an obstructing
> disease should be dispersed.[13]

Writing Down the Therapeutic Principles

This process of writing down exactly what is necessary to redress
the imbalance in theory is an indispensable part of the step by step
methodology I am advocating. It is the necessary intermediary step
which allows one to more clearly and easily deduce the required
treatment from the diagnosis. In Chinese TCM textbooks, it is said
that the therapeutic principles are the bridge between the diagnosis

---

[13] *Huang Di Nei Jing, Su Wen*, Chapter 74

and the treatment. Unfortunately, it is my experience that this step is almost always skipped by Western practitioners. By taking the time to consciously clarify what needs to be done in principle, the decision of how to do that becomes all the more obvious.

For instance, a 30 year old woman who had lost both her husband and son within the last year complained of early menstruation *(yue jing xian qi)* and excessive menstruation *(yue jing guo duo)*. Obviously she had experienced a great deal of mental and emotional anguish. Her periods had gradually become irregular and painful until becoming early and excessive. A bout of fever caused *beng* or avalanche bleeding after which she experienced unrelieved *lou* or trickle bleeding. Her face was pale, wan, and dull. She was exhausted and her spirit was *bu an*, not quiet. She complained of a dry mouth and thirst. Her menstrual discharge was bright red with purple clots. She experienced lower abdominal pain which was aggravated by pressure. Her tongue was pale red with a thin, white, *i.e.*, normal coating. Her pulse was wiry, fine, and fast.[14]

Analyzing the above signs and symptoms, we can conclude that this woman's mental and emotional stress had led to, on the one hand, heat as evidenced by her bleeding (heat causing the blood to flow recklessly outside its pathways), the bright red color of the discharge, her mental agitation (heat causing her spirit to be restless), and her red tongue and fast pulse. This disease dynamic is based on the dictum, "The five orientations (*i.e.*, emotions) transform into fire *(wu zhi hua huo)*." In this woman's case, this transformative fire from her emotions was then aggravated by an

---

[14] Excerpted from *Qian Jia Miao Fang (A Thousand Practitioners' Wondrous Prescriptions)*, Li Wan-liang, Qi Qiang, *et.al.*, Liberation Army Press, Beijing, 1985, trans. by Michael Helme and appearing in "Dysfunctional Uterine Bleeding" by Bob Flaws, *Free and Easy*, Blue Poppy Press, Boulder, CO, p. 75-76

acute febrile episode. On the other hand, her emotional stress had also seemingly caused stagnation of the qi and then eventually stasis of the blood. This is based on the idea that the qi commands the blood. This was evidenced by her dull complexion, lower abdominal pain aggravated by pressure, purple clots, by the fact that her *beng lou* had evolved from irregular and painful menstruation and by her wiry pulse. This disease dynamic is based on the liver storing the blood, the liver being the temperamental organ, and the liver qi governing the sea of blood. In addition, her wan, pale face, fatigue, pale tongue, and fine pulse plus her bleeding suggesting the qi being unable to hold the blood within its vessels all indicate qi vacuity.

According to the logic of Traditional Chinese Medicine, this woman's pattern discrimination is hot blood, qi vacuity, and stagnation and stasis of the qi and blood blocking her uterus. Therefore, the logical heteropathic therapeutic principles for the theoretic rectification of this woman's imbalance are to cool the blood and clear heat, boost the qi and fortify the spleen, quicken the blood and transform stasis. Based on these principles, it is a relatively simple matter to choose points which will catalyze these changes within the patient.

Stating Therapeutic Principles in the Correct Professional Terminology

As in the case of diagnosis, TCM has, over a period of two thousand years, worked out an agreed upon, time-tested list of therapeutic principles correlated to its professional diagnostic categories. In other words, one cannot capriciously list any therapeutic principle for any diagnostic pattern. There are specific principles that generations of practitioners have agreed upon as being the appropriate ones for specific patterns. For instance, clearing *(qing)* always means to clear heat. Therefore, if one clears the lungs or clears the blood, this implies that one is clearing some species of heat from the lungs or the blood.

In the first edition of this book, the Chinese *yi* was given as benefit. This erroneous translation does not mean anything in terms of the technical application of TCM. But when it is translated as boost, as in boost the qi, one knows immediately what technical intervention is meant. Likewise, in the first edition of this book, the Chinese word *li* was translated as facilitate. However, when it is translated as dinsinhibit, one knows immediately that the free flow of qi is inhibited in whatever part this word is coupled with and that treatment must free up this inhibition. Thus, disinhibiting the urination, the throat, the nose, etc. becomes intelligible in a technically precise way which the previous translation was not.

Below is a list of and a brief gloss on some of the most common TCM therapeutic principles abstracted from *Chinese-English Terminology of Traditional Chinese Medicine*.[15] Using this list, one can relatively easily move from deciding in principle what needs to be done to which points will, in fact, do this.

In emergency, treat the *biao* (branch symptoms); in chronic (cases), treat the *ben* (root cause). *(Ji ze zhi biao; han ze zhi ben.)*

Treat the *ben* and *biao* simultaneously. *(Biao ben tong zhi.)*

Support the righteous; eliminate evil. *(Fu zheng qu xie.)* This means to balance and support the patient's righteous qi at the same time as eliminating the evil qi.

---

[15] *Chinese-English Terminology of Traditional Chinese Medicine*, ed. by Sung J. Liao, Hunan Science and Technology Press, 1983, p. 330-402

Treat rightly. *(Zheng zhi.)* This means to treat heteropathically cold disease with warm methods and *vice versa*.

Treat contrarily. *(Fan zhi.)* This means to treat false cold with cold methods.

Treat below for diseases above. *(Shang bing xia zhi.)*

Treat above for diseases below. *(Xia bing shang zhi.)*

Treat yin in yang disease. *(Yang bing zhi yin.)* In acupuncture, this mainly refers to treating diseases of the yang channels via their *biao li* or external/internal paired yin channel.

Treat yang in yin disease. *(Yin bing zhi yang.)* Just the reverse of the above.

Treat yin if heat is aggravated by cold. *(Zhu han zhi er re zhe qu zhi yin.)* If a hot disease is worsened by cold therapy, supplement yin instead.

Treat yang if cold is aggravated by heat. *(Zhe re zhi er han zhe qu zhi yang.)* If a cold disease is worsened by heating therapy, supplement yang instead.

Invigorate the commander of water to counteract brilliant yang. *(Zhuang shui zhi zhu, yi zhi yang guang.)* For yang repletion, supplement the kidneys, *i.e.*, the commander of water.

Facilitate the source of fire to disperse excess yin. *(Yi huo zhi yang, yi xiao yin yi.)* Supplement kidney yang to transport, transport, and warm excessive dampness and cold.

Treat repletion by draining. *(Shi ze xie zhi.)*

Treat vacuity by supplementing. *(Xu ze bu zhi.)*

Treat heat by cooling. *(Re zhe han zhi.)* Literally, to treat heat with cold.

Treat cold by heating. *(Han zhe re zhi.)*

Treat guest (pathogens) by eliminating. *(Ke zhe chu zhi.)*

Mobilize the leisurely. *(Yi zhe xing zhi.)* This refers to quickening the retarded flow of qi and blood.

Treat retention by attacking. *(Liu zhe gong zhi.)* Retention implies retention of pathological substances, as in abdominal masses.

Treat dryness by moistening. *(Zhao zhe ru zhi.)*

Relax the tense. *(Ji zhe huan zhi.)* This means to relax spasmodic conditions.

Gather or restrain the scattered. *(San zhe shou zhi.)* This means to secure and astringe what has been excessively dispersed and effused.

Treat taxation by warming. *(Lao zhe wen zi.)* Warm supplementation should be used in cases of vacuity taxation.

Trim the hard. *(Jian zhe xue zhi.)* This means to reduce swellings and masses.

Raise the precipitated. *(Xia zhe ju zhi.)* This refers to treating prolapse of qi conditions by elevating the pure yang.

Suppress the risen. *(Gao zhe yi zhi.)* This refers to lowering upward counterflow.

Level fright. *(Jing zhe ping zhi.)* This means to level internally stirring wind in convulsive disorders.

Oppose the mild. *(Wei zhe ni zhi.)* This means to treat heteropathically mild conditions with consistent signs and symptoms, *i.e.*, mild cold diseases with cold symptoms should be warmed.

Follow the severe. *(Shen zhe cong zhi.)* Treat homeopathically severe conditions with false signs and symptoms according to the nature of those signs and symptoms, *i.e.*, severe hot diseases with cold symptoms should be cooled.

Enhance the mild. *(Yin qi qing er yang zhi.)* Treat mild external invasions by diaphoresis.

Reduce the severe. *(Yin qi zhong er jian zhi.)* Treat serious internal pathogens by purging and dispersing.

Strengthen the debilitated. *(Yin qi shuai er zhang zhi.)* When the virulence of the evil qi is on the wane but the righteous qi has not recuperated, supplement the righteous rather than further attacking evil.

Vault the high. *(Qi gao zhe yin er yue zhi.)* Induce vomiting.

Lead away and cleanse those (pathogens) in the lower (burner). *(Qi xia zhe yin er jie zhi.)* This refers to precipitation (*i.e.*, purgation of the bowels) and diuresis.

Do not sweat in blood loss; do not bleed in excessive sweating. *(Duo xue zhe wu han, duo han zhe wu xue.)*

For fullness in the middle, purge the inside. *(Zhong man zhe, xie zhi yu nei.)* This refers to treating abdominal distention through precipitation.

Do not damage with heat in heat. *(Re wu fan re.)* This means to be careful using warming methods in the summer.

Do not damage with cold in cold. *(Han wu fan han.)* Be careful using cooling methods in the winter.

Do not damage the stomach qi. *(Wu fan wei qi.)* Care should be taken to protect the stomach qi which is the root of postnatal qi or acquired essence.

Ou-thrust depressed wood. *(Mu yu da zhi.)* This means to rectify the qi and resolve depression by using qi-moving, exterior-relieving methods.

Effuse depressed fire. *(Huo yu fa zhi.)* For internal heat and *no* sweating, diaphoresis can be used.

Drain depressed metal. *(Jin yu xie zhi.)* This refers to draining stagnant lung qi.

Retrench depressed earth. *(Tu yu duo zhi.)* This means to eliminate stagnant dampness from the middle.

Regulate depressed water. *(Shui yu zhe zhi.)* This means to drain stagnant water by promoting urination.

In vacuity, supplement the mother. *(Xu zhe bu qi mu.)* This refers to supplementation according to the *sheng* cycle of the five phases.

In repletion, drain the child. *(Shi zhe xie qi zi.)* This refers to draining repletion according to the *sheng* cycle.

Relieve or resolve the exterior. *(Jie biao.)*

Relieve the muscles. *(Jie ji.)* This means to sweat out external pathogens in the muscles and the skin.

Dissipate the exterior. *(Shu biao.)*

Out-thrust rashes. *(Tou zhen.)* This means to facilitate the eruption of a rash.

Out-thrust macules. *(Tou ban.)* This means to use exterior-relieving medicinals to facilitate the resolution of purpuric macules.

Out-thrust evils. *(Tou xie.)* This refers to sweating out pathogens from the exterior.

Out-thrust the exterior. *(Tou biao.)* **Same as above.**

Course wind. *(Shu feng.)* This also means to sweat out evil wind from the exterior.

Out-thrust wind and exteriorize heat. *(Tou feng yu re wai.)*

Out-thrust and discharge. *(Tou xie.)* This means to both relieve the exterior and simultaneously to precipitate the interior.

Open the devils' gates. *(Kai gui men.)* To induce perspiration. The devils' gates is another name for the *qi men* or pores.

Nourish yin and relieve the exterior. *(Yang yin jie biao.)*

Boost the qi and relieve the exterior. *(Yi qi jie biao.)*

Support the yang and relieve the exterior. *(Zhu yang jie biao.)*

Nourish the blood and relieve the exterior. *(Yang xue jie biao.)*

Transform rheum and relieve the exterior. *(Hua yin jie biao.)*

Relieve simultaneously the exterior and interior. *(Biao li shuang jie.)* This is another way to describe using both precipitation and diaphoresis together.

Open and raise. *(Kai ti.)* This refers to simultaneously relieving the exterior and raising the clear qi in cases of diarrhea due to internal invasion with exterior symptoms.

Discharge heat through the defensive. *(Xie wei tou re.)* This means to resolve the exterior and thus discharge heat in the case of a *wei fen* warm disease.

Clear the qi. *(Qing qi.)* This means to clear heat from the *qi fen* or qi division.

Engender fluids. *(Sheng jin.)* This means to catalyze the generation of body fluids.

Boost the qi and engender fluids. *(Yi qi sheng jin.)*

Clear and discharge the *shao yang*. *(Qing xie shao yang.)*

Clear heat and resolve toxins. *(Qing re jie du.)*

Clear heat and resolve summerheat. *(Qing re jie shu.)*

Clear the *ying*. *(Qing ying.)* This means to clear heat from the *ying fen* or constructive division in the case of a warm disease.

Clear the heart. *(Qing xin.)* To clear heat from the heart.

Clear both the qi and *ying*. *(Qi ying liang qing.)* To clear heat from both the qi and constructive divisions simultaneously.

Clear the constructive and out-thrust rashes. *(Qing ying tou zhen.)*

Cool the blood. *(Liang xue.)*

Cool the blood and resolve toxins. *(Liang xue jie du.)*

Drain the heart. *(Xie xin.)* This means to drain pathologic heat from the heart.

Discharge and precipitate. *(Xie xia.)* This refers to purgation through intestinal catharsis.

Increase humors, discharge and precipitate. *(Zeng ye xie xia.)*

Supplement and attack simultaneously. *(Gong bu jian shi.)* To simultaneously supplement the righteous and attack the pathologic.

Attack first and then supplement. *(Xian gong hou bu.)* To attack evil before supplementing the righteous.

Supplement first and then attack. *(Xian bu hou gong.)* To supplement the righteous first and then to attack the evil qi.

31

Eliminate stale water. *(Qu wan chen cuo.)* This means to remove old pathological products, such as edema and static blood.

Free the bowels and discharge heat. *(Tong fu xie re.)*

Abduct stagnation and free the bowels. *(Dao zhi tong fu.)* This includes stagnations of heat, blood stasis, and water.

Urgently precipitate to preserve yin. *(Ji xia cun yin.)* This refers to precipitating in a timely manner in internal heat diseases so as to protect yin fluids.

Rake the firewood from under the cauldron. *(Fu di chou xin.)* This means to precipitate replete heat from the bowels to dissipate the cause of the accumulation of heat.

Harmonize and resolve the *shao yang. (He jie shao yang.)* To harmonize and resolve the internal and the external in a half-internal/half-external *shan han bing* where there is alternating fever and chills.

Regulate and harmonize the liver and spleen. *(Tiao he gan pi.)*

Regulate and harmonize the liver and stomach. *(Tiao he gan wei.)*

Dispel dampness. *(Qu shi.)*

Transform dampness. *(Hua shi.)*

Dry dampness. *(Zao shi.)*

Disinhibit dampness. *(Li shi.)*

Clear heat and disinhibit dampness. *(Qing re li shi.)*

Clear summerheat and disinhibit dampness. *(Qing shu li shi.)*

Warm yang and disinhibit dampness. *(Wen yang li shi.)*

Enrich yin and disinhibit dampness. *(Zi yin li shi.)*

Warm the kidneys and disinhibit water. *(Wen shen li shui.)*

Percolate dampness through the heat. *(Shen shi yu re xia.)* This refers to excreting evil dampness in order to precipitate heat in cases of damp heat where dampness is more serious than heat.

Disinhibit the urination (to treat) repletion of the stools. *(Li xiao bian, shi da bian.)* This means to induce urination in order to treat damp heat diarrhea.

Fortify the spleen. *(Jian pi.)*

Transport or move the spleen. *(Yun pi.)* This means to mobilize the spleen's transportation of body fluids so as to eliminate dampness.

Bank earth. *(Bei tu.)* To supplement the spleen.

Bank earth to engender metal. *(Bei tu sheng jin.)* This means to supplement earth so as to engender the lungs.

Fortify the spleen and course the liver. *(Jian pi shu gan.)*

Supplement the spleen and boost the lungs. *(Bu pi yi fei.)*

Warm and supplement the *ming men*. *(Wen bu ming men.)*

Course the liver. *(Shu gan.)* This means to rectify the qi of the liver in case of depression and stagnation.

Soften the liver. *(Rou gan.)* This implies nourishing liver blood.

Inhibit the liver. *(Fa gan.)* This is a method of draining used in cases of hyperactivity of the liver.

Enrich and nourish the liver and kidneys. *(Zi yang gan shen.)* This means to nourish liver blood and enrich kidney yin.

Harmonize the liver. *(He gan.)* This means to nourish liver blood at the same time as coursing the liver and rectifying the qi.

Enrich yin, level the liver, and subdue yang. *(Zi yin, ping gan, qian yang.)*

Draining the liver. *(Xie gan.)* To drain repletion from the liver.

Help metal to level wood. *(Zuo jin ping mu.)* This means to clear and depurate the lungs so that the lungs can restrain the liver via the *ke* cycle of the five phases.

Enrich yin. *(Zi yin.)*

Protect the yin by clearing the connecting vessels. *(Qing luo bao yin.)* To clear heat from the connecting vessels in order to protect yin from scorching and consumption.

Harden yin. *(Jian yin.)* This means to clear heat and secure kidney essence.

Strengthen yin. *(Qiang yin.)* To supplement and boost yin essence.

Constrain yin. *(Lian yin.)* To treat dissipation of yin fluids by astringing.

Subdue yang. *(Qian yang.)* To subdue hyperactivity of liver yang.

Subdue and settle. *(Qian zhen.)* This means to subdue and settle upward hyperactivity of liver yang and internal wind.

Extinguish wind. *(Xi feng.)* This is a collective term for extinguishing specifically stirring of internal wind. The specific methods of accomplishing this depending on the disease dynamic responsible for the wind are given below.

Enrich yin and extinguish wind. *(Zi yin xi feng.)*

Level the liver and extinguish wind. *(Ping gan xi feng.)*

Drain fire and extinguish wind. *(Xie huo xi feng.)*

Harmonize the blood and extinguish wind. *(He xue xi feng.)*

Relieve or resolve fright. *(Jie jing.)* This means to relieve or resolve spasms and convulsions.

Dispel wind. *(Qu feng.)* This refers to treating external wind manifesting as musculoskeletal problems, *i.e.*, to search out wind and treat it in the skin, channels, muscles, and joints.

Dispel wind and eliminate dampness. *(Qu feng qu shi.)* To treat wind dampness or rheumatic conditions.

Course wind and discharge heat. *(Shu feng xie re.)* This means to treat external wind combined with internal heat.

Dispel wind and nourish the blood. *(Qu feng yang xue.)*

Track (down) wind and dispel cold. *(Sou feng zhu han.)*

Moisten dryness. *(Run zao.)*

Clear and diffuse (the lungs) and moisten dryness. *(Qing xuan run zao.)*

Clear the intestines and moisten dryness. *(Qing chang run zao.)*

Nourish yin and moisten dryness. *(Yang yin run zao.)*

Nourish the blood and moisten dryness. *(Yang xue run zao.)*

Rectify the qi. *(Li qi.)*

Course the liver and rectify the qi. *(Shu gan li qi.)*

Harmonize the stomach and rectify the qi. *(He wei li qi.)*

Descend or precipitate the qi. *(Xia qi.)* As in cases of upward counterflow.

Regulate the qi. *(Tiao qi.)*

Break the qi. *(Po qi.)* To strongly crack or break qi stagnation.

Expel phlegm. *(Qu tan.)* To cause expectoration.

Transform phlegm. *(Hua tan.)*

Diffuse the lungs and transform phlegm. *(Xuan fei hua tan.)*

Clear heat and transform phlegm. *(Qing re hua tan.)*

Moisten the lungs and transform phlegm. *(Run fei hua tan.)*

Dry dampness and transform phlegm. *(Zao shi hua tan.)*

Dispel cold and transform phlegm. *(Qu han hua tan.)*

Treat wind and transform phlegm. *(Zhi feng hua tan.)*

Disperse phlegm. *(Xiao tan.)* Specifically, stagnant phlegm.

Diffuse the lungs. *(Xuan fei.)*

Clear the lungs and perdure the qi. *(Qing fei su qi.)* This refers to clearing heat from the lungs and regulating counterflowing lung qi.

Draining the lungs. *(Xie fei.)* To drain repletion from the lungs.

Diffuse and open the water passageways. *(Xuan tong shui dao.)* This principle is applied in the treatment of lung edema where an external evil is obstructing the downward diffusion of lung qi and, therefore, the lung's function of sending water downward to be excreted with urination.

Nourish the yin and clear the lungs. *(Yang yin qing fei.)*

Treat the lungs and kidneys simultaneously. *(Fei shen tong zhi.)*

Soften the hard and scatter nodulation. *(Ruan jian san jie.)* This means to treat hard, nodular swellings and masses due to accumulation and gathering of phlegm and static blood.

Rectify the blood. *(Li xue.)*

Warm the blood. *(Wen xue.)*

Dispel stasis and quicken the blood. *(Qu yu huo xue.)*

Quicken the blood and dispel stasis. *(Huo xue qu yu.)*

Break stasis and disperse swelling. *(Po yu xiao zhong.)*

Dispel stasis and disperse swelling. *(Qu yu xiao zhong.)*

Break the blood. *(Po xue.)* To crack substantial blood stasis.

Stop bleeding. *(Zhi xue.)*

Clear heat and stop bleeding. *(Qing re zhi xue.)*

Supplement the qi and stop bleeding. *(Bu qi zhi xue.)*

Dispel stasis and stop bleeding. *(Qu yu zhi xue.)*

Open the portals. *(Kai qiao.)*

Clear heat and open the portals. *(Qing re kai qiao.)*

Clear heat, transform phlegm, and open the portals. *(Qing re, hua tan, kai qiao.)*

Dispel cold and open the portals. *(Zhu han kai qiao.)*

Transform phlegm and open the portals. *(Hua tan kai qiao.)*

Eject phlegm and arouse the brain. *(Yong tan xing nao.)*

Return yang and stem counterflow. *(Hui yang jiu ni.)*

Warm the middle and dispel cold. *(Wen zhong qu han.)*

Warm the channels and scatter cold. *(Wen jing san han.)*

Warm the yang. *(Wen yang.)*

Free yang. *(Tong yang.)*

Warm the spleen. *(Wen pi.)*

Rectify the middle. *(Li zhong.)*

Stem desertion. *(Jiu tuo.)*

Free the vessels. *(Tong mai.)*

Harmonize the middle. *(He zhong.)*

Quiet the middle. *(An zhong.)*

Harmonize the stomach. *(He wei.)*

Boost the stomach. *(Yi wei.)* This means to supplement stomach qi.

Warm the stomach and fortify the middle. *(Wen wei jian zhong.)*

Enrich and nourish stomach yin. *(Zi yang wei yin.)*

Disperse food and abduct stagnation. *(Xiao shi dao zhi.)*

Disperse glomus. *(Xiao pi.)*

Open glomus. *(Kai pi.)*

Open the stomach. *(Kai wei.)*

Terminate malaria. *(Jie Nue.)* *Nue* is usually translated as malaria, and malarial episodes can be prevented by timely acupuncture.

Supplement yin. *(Bu yin.)*

Supplement yang. *(Bu yang.)*

Invigorate yang. *(Zhuang yang.)*

Supplement the qi. *(Bu qi.)*

Upbear and raise the middle qi. *(Sheng ti zhong qi.)* As in cases of fall of the middle qi.

Supplement the qi and secure the exterior. *(Bu qi gu biao.)* This means to supplement the defensive qi and to close the pores.

Boost the qi and engender fluids. *(Yi qi sheng jin.)*

Supplement the blood. *(Bu xue.)*

Quiet the spirit. *(An shen.)*

Constrain perspiration and secure the exterior. *(Lian han gu biao.)*

Constrain the lungs and stop coughing. *(Lian fei zhi ke.)*

40

Astringe the intestines and stop diarrhea. *(Se chang zhi xie.)*

Secure the kidneys and astringe the essence. *(Gu shen se jing.)*

Secure *beng* and stop dai. *(Gu beng zhi dai.)* *Beng* means excessive uterine bleeding. *Dai* means abnormal vaginal discharge.

Supplement the kidneys. *(Bu shen.)*

Warm the kidneys. *(Wen shen.)*

Enrich the kidneys. *(Zi shen.)* This means to enrich kidney yin.

Supplement the kidneys to grasp the qi. *(Bu shen na qi.)* This refers to the respiratory qi sent down to the kidneys by the lungs.

Guide fire back to its source. *(Yin huo gui yuan.)* This means to lead vacuity fire back down to the lower burner.

(Maintain) communication between the heart and kidneys. *(Jiao tong xin shen.)* As in cases of heart fire above and kidney yin vacuity below.

Regulate menstruation. *(Tiao jing.)*

Free menstruation. *(Tong jing.)* This means to induce the period if it is overdue or absent.

Promote lactation. *(Cui ru.)*

Evacuate pus and expel toxins. *(Pai nong tuo du.)*

Expel worms. *(Qu chong.)*

Of the above approximately 230 traditional Chinese therapeutic principles, a number are synonymous. In Chinese, one might pick one construction over another purely based on whether its sound in combination with other principles were harmonious. For instance, *zi yin* and *yang yin* both mean to nourish the yin. Other principles, such as *he gan*, to harmonize the liver, appear at first to have only a general meaning, but in fact, in TCM mean something quite specific although not explicitly stated. In this case, *he gan* implies nourishing the blood while at the same time regulating the flow of stagnant liver qi. Whereas, in the case of *he wei* or *he zhong*, to harmonize the stomach or middle (burner), harmonizing here merely implies regulation of the stomach qi with upbearing of the pure and downbearing of the turbid with the emphasis on descending upwardly counterflowing stomach qi. Therefore, the student is advised to pay close attention to the implied Chinese meaning of these treatment principles as they appear in the literature.

It is my hope that, by making this list of traditional treatment principles more readily available to Western practitioners, more English-speaking practitioners will routinely include the conscious formulation of such principles in their process. This step is routinely taught at Chinese TCM colleges, is routinely applied in Chinese TCM clinics, and routinely appears in the vast majority of contemporary Chinese TCM treatment-oriented literature. Although some may disagree with some of the above translations, I nevertheless hope that more attention will be given to the correct formulation of therapeutic principles in the West in the future.

To reiterate this process, if a patient's TCM pattern diagnosis is insomnia and palpitations due to heart (blood) and spleen (qi) dual vacuity (*xin pi liang xu*), and if one knows that, according to TCM heteropathy, one needs to nourish heart blood, supplement spleen qi, and quiet the spirit, then it is a relatively simple task to choose points which will accomplish these principles. In the following chapter are lists of the major TCM therapeutic functions of the most important acupuncture points and their most common combinations, thus making the co-ordination of the above principles with specific points all the easier.

4

Choosing Points Based on Principle (1)

H aving stated in principle what needs to be done in order to rebalance or rectify a patient's situation, next the practitioner must erect a treatment plan which rationally implements each of these therapeutic principles. Having previously clarified what in principle needs to be done, one selects points which will, in fact, do what is required.

Below is a list of the most commonly used acupuncture points with their main TCM functions stated in terms of the foregoing treatment principles. This is then followed by a list of the most common two and three point combinations and their TCM functions. I have composed these lists based on lecture notes from Dr. Xi Yang-jiang of the Shanghai College of Traditional Chinese Medicine[16] and on the traditional functions for points given in *Acupuncture: A Comprehensive Text*[17] and *Fundamentals of Chinese Acupuncture*.[18]

---

[16] Xi Yang-jiang, lecture notes from an acupuncture seminar given in San Francisco, 1983, under the auspices of the American Foundation of Traditional Chinese Medicine

[17] Shanghai College of Traditional Chinese Medicine, *Acupuncture: A Comprehensive Text*, trans. and ed. by John O'Connor and Dan Bensky, Eastland Press, Chicago, 1981

[18] Ellis, Andrew; Wiseman, Nigel; and Boss, Ken; *Fundamentals of Chinese Acupuncture*, Paradigm Publications, Brookline, MA, 1988

Following these two lists is a recapitulation of the same material but working from the opposite direction. This is a list of the main therapeutic functions and the most common acupuncture points which fulfill these functions. This list has been translated from *Zhong Guo Zhen Jiu Chu Fang Xue (The Theory of Writing Prescriptions in Chinese Acupuncture/Moxibustion).*

Working from these lists, one should be able to logically select the several main or commanding points *(zhu xue)* of their acupuncture formula which will accomplish their stated treatment goals. These commanding points should then be supplemented by one or more local points of appropriate symptomatic action. These are called the adjunctive or supplementary points *(bei xue).*

Functions of Individual Major Acupoints

Hand *Tai Yin* Lung Channel

Zhong Fu (Lu 1) Regulates and rectifies the lung qi
　　　　　　　Nourishes lung yin
　　　　　　　Clears heat from the upper burner

Yun Men (Lu 2) Rectifies the lungs
　　　　　　　Transforms phlegm
　　　　　　　Clears lung heat and eliminates vexation

Chi Ze (Lu 5)　Rectifies the lung qi
　　　　　　　Normalizes counterflow qi
　　　　　　　Clears heat from lungs and eliminates vexation
　　　　　　　Clears heat from the upper burner
　　　　　　　He sea point of the lungs

Lie Que (Lu 7) Diffuses the lung qi
　　　　　　　Expels wind, scatters cold

Relieves the exterior
Disinhibits urination by downbearing the turbid
Clears and regulates the *ren mai*
Luo point of the hand *tai yin*
Hui meeting point of the *ren mai*

Tai Yuan (Lu 9) Clears heat
Dispels wind
Transforms phlegm
Rectifies the lung qi
Downbears and depurates the lung qi
Clears heat from the upper burner
Diffuses the lung qi
Stops coughing
Yuan source point of the lungs

Shao Shang (Lu 11)
Clears heat from the lungs
Disinhibits the throat
Dispels wind, as in convulsions
Revives from loss of consciousness due to
heatstroke

Hand *Yang Ming* Large Intestine Channel

He Gu (LI 4) Clears heat from the *qi fen*
Clears heat from the portals of the head
and face
Expels wind
Relieves the exterior
Upbears the clear and downbears the turbid
Diffuses the lung qi
Reduces fever
Frees the flow of the channels

47

Stops pain
Scatters cold
Opens the bowels
Yuan source point of the hand *yang ming*

Qu Chi (LI 11) Dispels wind and clears heat
Protects fluids and humors
Clears heat from the blood
Eliminates dampness
Harmonizes the qi and blood
Rectifies the blood
Rectifies the lung qi
Relieves the exterior

Jian Yu (LI 15) Dispels evil wind from the four extremities
Disinhibits the joints
Harmonizes the qi and blood
Opens the connecting vessels

Ying Xiang (LI 20)
Clears wind heat from the *yang ming*
Dispels wind heat from the exterior
Disinhibits the nasal passages
Confluent point of hand and foot *yang ming*

Foot *Yang Ming* Stomach Channel

Di Cang (St 4) Frees the flow of qi in the channels of the face
Confluent point of the hand and foot *yang ming*,
ren, and *qiao* channels

Liang Men (St 21)
Promotes the transportation and transformation of
grain and liquids

Disperses stagnant food
Rectifies the center
Harmonizes the stomach and intestines
Fortifies the spleen

Tian Shu (St 25) Moves the qi
Upbears the clear and downbears the turbid
Opens the bowels
Transforms dampness
Banks earth
Clears heat from the large intestine
Front *mu* point of the large intestine

Shui Dao (St 28)
Rectifies the qi of the triple heater and bladder
Disinhibits urination and percolates water
  dampness
Clears and eliminates damp heat
Frees the flow in the lower burner

Gui Lai (St 29) Frees the flow of the qi and blood of the lower
  burner
Dispels stasis
Warms the uterus
Stops pain

Liang Qiu (St 34)
Clears heat from the stomach
Harmonizes the stomach and descends counterflow
Dispels stasis and accumulation in the *yang ming*
Clears the channels and quickens the connecting
  vessels
Xi cleft point of the foot yang ming

Zu San Li (St 36)

Fortifies the spleen
Boosts the lungs so as to resist external invasion
Rectifies upbearing of the clear and downbearing
   of the turbid
Descends counterflow qi
Stops vomiting
Disperses food stagnation
Breaks blood stasis in the chest
Dries and eliminates dampness
Harmonizes the spleen and stomach
Supplements vacuity
Supports the righteous and secures the root
Rectifies the qi and blood
Clears heat from the six bowels
He sea point of the foot *yang ming*

Feng Long (St 40)

Discharges heat of the stomach and small intestine
Harmonizes the spleen and stomach
Transforms phlegm and eliminates dampness
Opens the portals of the heart when misted by
   phlegm
Downbears the turbid
Luo point of the foot *yang ming*

Jie Xi (St 41)
Clears and discharges fire
Clears heat from the stomach
Transforms dampness and stasis
Quiets the spirit

Chong Yang (St 42)

Drains replete fire of the *yang ming*
Banks earth
Transforms dampness

Harmonizes the stomach
Quiets the spirit

Nei Ting (St 44) Clears heat from the stomach
Opens the bowels
Harmonizes the stomach
Downbears the turbid
Normalizes counterflow qi
Stops pain, especially abdominal pain with fever

Foot *Tai Yin* Spleen Channel

Yin Bai (Sp 1)   Rectifies the qi of the spleen channel
Warms the spleen and invigorates yang
Dispels cold from the middle and lower burners
Boosts the qi to facilitate the spleen's holding the
   blood within its channels
Clears the heart
Quiets the spirit
Jing well point of the foot *tai yin*

Gong Sun (Sp 4)
Rectifies the qi of the middle burner
Descends counterflow qi
Downbears the turbid
Dispels cold from the heart and abdomen
Harmonizes the *chong mai*
Regulates the sea of blood
Rectifies the qi dynamic
Supports the spleen and stomach
Luo point of the foot *tai yin*
Hui meeting point of the *chong mai*

51

San Yin Jiao (Sp 6)

Fortifies the spleen
Eliminates dampness
Enriches yin
Nourishes the blood
Rectifies the blood
Transforms blood stasis
Warms the middle and lower burners
Dispels cold from the blood
Regulates the blood chamber and the palace of essence
Moves the qi
Aids transportation and transformation
Subdues liver heat
Courses liver qi
Boosts the kidneys
Confluent point of the three leg yin

Di Ji (Sp 8)

Rectifies the qi of the spleen channel
Moves and quickens the qi and blood
Harmonizes the blood
Regulates the uterus
Xi cleft point of foot *tai yin*

Yin Ling Quan (Sp 9)

Warms and moves the middle burner
Transforms and resolves depressive dampness
Disinhibits the lower burner
Fortifies the spleen
Transforms and eliminates phlegm and dampness
Disinhibits urination and opens the water passageways
Clears and eliminates dampness and heat
He sea point of the foot *tai yin*

Xue Hai (Sp 10)Rectifies and clears the blood
Moves the lower burner

Hand *Shao Yin* Heart Channel

Tong Li (Ht 5)   Clears heat from the heart
Opens the portals of the heart
Quiets the spirit
Rectifies heart qi
Luo point of the heart channel

Shen Men (Ht 7) Clears the heart
Clears fire and cools the *ying*
Quiets the spirit and tranquilizes the heart
Moves the qi and dispels stasis from the heart
Opens the channels (of the chest) and moves *bi*
Yuan source and *shu* stream point of the heart
channel

Hand *Tai Yang* Small Intestine Channel

Shao Ze (SI 1)   Clears heat from the small intestine
Dispels obstruction from the channels of the
breast
Promotes lactation
Clears heart fire
Out-thrusts depressive heat
Dispels wind and clears heat
Jing well point of the hand *tai yang*

Hou Xi (SI 3)   Disperses heat from the exterior
Relaxes the sinews
Secures the exterior

Out-thrusts internal heat
Opens the *du mai*
Clears the heart spirit
Hui meeting point of the *du mai*
Shu stream point of the hand *tai yang*

Foot *Tai Yang* Bladder Channel

Jing Ming (Bl 1)

Dispels wind
Clears heat
Opens the channels
Brightens the eyes
Enriches water (*vis à vis* the eyes)
Confluent point of stomach, triple heater, *yang*
and *yin qiao mai,* and bladder channels

Zan Zhu (Bl 2)   Dispels wind
Supplements kidney water (*vis à vis* the eyes)
Nourishes liver wood (*vis à vis* the eyes)
Disinhibits lacrimation
Brightens the eyes

Tian Zhu (Bl 10)

Free the flow of the channels of the neck
Dispels wind and scatters cold
Soothes the sinews
Opens the connecting vessels
Clears the head
Brightens the eyes
Clears fire
Descends counterflow qi
Window of the sky point

Da Shu (Bl 11) Frees the flow of the *tai yang* in the upper back
        Dispels evil wind
        Relieves external heat
        Soothes the sinews and vessels
        Hui meeting point of the bones

Feng Men (Bl 12)
        Dispels wind and eliminates dampness
        Relieves the exterior
        Diffuses the lung qi
        Transforms phlegm
        Rectifies the lung qi

Fei Shu (Bl 13) Frees the flow of lungs qi
        Rectifies the lung qi
        Clears heat from the lungs
        Clears vacuity heat from the lungs
        Harmonizes the *ying* and blood
        Stops coughing
        Back *shu* point of the lungs

Xin Shu (Bl 15) Supplements the heart qi
        Nourishes heart blood
        Clears heart fire
        Removes obstruction from the heart
        Rectifies the qi and blood
        Quiets the spirit
        Loosens the chest
        Back *shu* point of the heart

Ge Shu (Bl 17) Rectifies the blood
        Transforms blood stasis
        Clears heat from the blood
        Expands the chest and diaphragm
        Strengthens vacuity conditions

Harmonizes stomach qi

Hui meeting point of the blood

Gan Shu (Bl 18)

Harmonizes the liver

Resolves liver depression

Disinhibits the liver and gallbladder

Nourishes (liver) blood and *ying*

Clears and eliminates damp heat from the liver and gallbladder

Brightens the eyes

Quiets the spirit

Back *shu* point of the liver

Pi Shu (Bl 20) Rectifies the spleen qi

Promotes transportation and transformation of fluids

Eliminates dampness

Harmonizes the blood

Boosts the qi

Back *shu* point of the spleen

Wei Shu (Bl 21)

Rectifies the center and harmonizes the stomach

Transforms dampness

Eliminates stagnation

Banks the *yuan* original qi

Supplements the middle (burner)

Back *shu* point of the stomach

Shen Shu (Bl 23)

Boosts kidney qi

Supplements the kidneys

Enriches water

Boosts water and invigorates fire

Strengthens *qi hua* (kidney qi transformation of
water)
Disinhibits water dampness
Subdues liver fire
Rectifies the kidney qi
Strengthens the lumbus
Brightens the eyes and sharpens the hearing
Back *shu* point of the kidneys

Da Chang Shu (Bl 25)

Rectifies conveyance and conduction of large
intestine
Rectifies the qi and transforms stasis
Back *shu* point of the large intestine

Xiao Chang Shu (Bl 27)

Promotes the separation of the clear and turbid
Disinhibits urination
Percolates dampness
Transforms gatherings and accumulations
Opens and rectifies the small intestine
Clears heat from the intestines
Back *shu* point of the small intestine

Pang Guang Shu (Bl 28)

Rectifies the bladder qi
Disinhibits the low back
Dispels wind and eliminates dampness
Supplements the lower origin
Disinhibits urination
Clears heat
Back *shu* point of bladder

Wei Zhong (Bl 40)

Drains summerheat

57

Disinhibits the low back and knees
Clears heat from the blood
Frees the flow of the channels and connecting
vessels
Soothes the sinews and frees the connecting
vessels
He sea point of the foot *tai yang*

Gao Huang Shu (Bl 43)
Rectifies the lung qi
Supplements the heart qi
Supplements the lungs and fortifies the spleen
Tranquilizes the heart and banks the kidneys
Clears vacuity heat
Descends counterflow qi
Transforms phlegm
Supplements vacuity conditions

Zhi Shi (Bl 52) Secures the essence
Supplements the *zhen yin* or true yin
Supplements the kidneys and fulfills the essence
Disinhibits urination and percolates dampness

Kun Lun (Bl 60)
Promotes qi transformation of liquids
Downbears the turbid
Quickens the blood
Dispels pathogens from the *tai yang*
Dispels blood stasis in the uterus
Soothes the sinews and transforms dampness
Strengthens the kidneys and lumbus

Shen Mai (Bl 62)
Quiets the spirit

Soothes the channel sinews
Hui meeting point of the *yang qiao mai*
Expels external pathogens from the exterior
Treats wind diseases
Quiets the spirit

Zhi Yin (Bl 67) Eliminates dampness
Percolates dampness
Clears the brain above
Regulates pregnancy and childbirth below
Rectifies the qi and quickens the blood
Courses wind in the vertex
Brightens the eyes
Jing well point of the foot *tai yang*

Foot *Shao Yin* Kidney Channel

Yong Quan (Ki 1)
Supplements the kidneys
Fulfills the essence
Enriches yin
Enriches yin so as to control ministerial fire
Enriches kidney water so as to subdue liver fire
Descends upwardly-rising fire
Opens the portals for resuscitation
Quiets the spirit

Tai Xi (Ki 3)   Boosts kidney water and clears its source
Rectifies the qi of the kidney channel
Enriches the kidneys
Descends fire
Supplements the kidneys
Nourishes yin so as to moisten the lungs
Abates vacuity heat

Regulates the uterus
Invigorates source yang
Strengthens the lower back and knees

Da Zhong (Ki 4)
Supplements the kidneys
Boosts the essence so as to brighten the mind
Luo point of the foot *shao yin*

Zhao Hai (Ki 6) Eliminates dampness
Boosts the kidneys
Rectifies the qi of the kidney channel
Induces vacuity fire downward
Leads yin upward so as to boost the qi
Clears heat
Quiets the spirit
Disinhibits the throat
Hui meeting point of the *yin qiao mai*

Fu Liu (Ki 7) Rectifies the qi of the kidney channel
Clears heat
Eliminates dampness
Secures the defensive qi
Regulates the pores
Disinhibits the bladder
Moistens dryness
Enriches the kidneys
Jing river point of foot *shao yin*

Shu Fu (Ki 27) Descends counterflow qi
Rectifies the lung qi
Stabilizes wheezing
Stops coughing
Fortifies the spleen and harmonizes the stomach

Hand *Jue Yin* Pericardium Channel

Tian Chi (Per 1) Removes obstruction of qi flow in the *jue yin*
Confluent point of hand and foot *jue yin* and foot
shao yin
Loosens the chest and rectifies the qi
Stabilizes wheezing
Stops coughing
Diffuses the lungs
Clears heat

Xi Men (Per 4) Tranquilizes the heart
Quiets the spirit
Rectifies the qi
Clears the *ying*
Cools the blood
Loosens the diaphragm
Stops palpitations
Xi cleft point of the hand *jue yin*

Jian Shi (Per 5) Quiets the spirit
Harmonizes the stomach
Transforms phlegm
Clears the heart
Loosens the chest
Soothes the sinews
Quickens the connecting vessels
Nourishes the heart
Resolves depression so as to clear the pericardium
Jing river point of the hand *jue yin*

Nei Guan (Per 6)
Tranquilizes the heart
Calms the mind
Rectifies the qi

Stops pain
Diffuses the qi and promotes the qi function of the
upper and middle burners
Descends counterflow qi
Loosens the chest and expands the diaphragm
Clears the heart
Clears heat
Harmonizes the stomach and stops vomiting
Resolves depression of the liver
Resolves depression of the epigastrium
Luo point of the hand *jue yin*
Hui meeting point of the *yin wei mai*

Da Ling (Per 7) Clears and discharges heart fire
Dispels the evil qi of the heart and chest
Quiets the spirit
Clears the *ying* and cools the blood
Harmonizes the stomach
Loosens the chest
Shu stream point and *yuan* source point of the
hand *jue yin*

Lao Gong (Per 8)
Clears the pericardium
Clears heart fire
Discharges evil heat to resuscitate
Clear and eliminates damp heat
Quiets the spirit
Harmonizes the stomach
Extinguishes wind
Cools the blood
Rong spring point of hand *jue yin*

Hand *Shao Yang* Triple Heater Channel

Guan Chong (TH 1)

Clears heat from the large intestine and triple heater channels

Out-thrusts and effuses heat accumulation of the triple heater channel

Dispels wind and disperses evil

Clears heat and drains fire

Jing well point of the hand *shao yang*

Wai Guan (TH 5)

Relieves the exterior

Disperses wind

Clears heat and resolves toxins

Frees the flow qi in the channels

Luo point of the hand *shao yang*

Hui meeting point of the *yang wei mai*

Zhi Gou (TH 6)

Resolves depressive fire of the triple heater

Diffuses the qi

Downbears counterflow and fire

Disperses obstruction

Opens the intestines

Frees the bowel qi

Tian Jing (TH 10)

Rectifies the qi of the triple heater channel

Transforms phlegm dampness in the channels and connecting vessels

Courses fire qi in the triple heater

He sea point of the hand *shao yang*

Yi Feng (TH 17)
>>> Expels wind
>>> Clears heat
>>> Frees the flow of the channels
>>> Relieves spasms
>>> Disinhibits hearing and vision
>>> Opens the portals

Foot *Shao Yang* Gallbladder Channel

Feng Chi (GB 20)
>>> Expels (external) wind
>>> Clears heat
>>> Disperses (internal) wind
>>> Discharges liver fire
>>> Settles (internal) wind
>>> Dispels wind heat
>>> Harmonizes the qi and blood
>>> Clears the head and opens the portals
>>> Frees the channels and quickens the connecting vessels
>>> Disinhibits the hearing and vision

Jian Jing (GB 21)
>>> Disperses wood qi
>>> Frees the flow of the qi in the *yang ming* channel traversing the breast
>>> Clears heat
>>> Disperses stagnation
>>> Stops pain
>>> Expels retained placenta
>>> Frees the channels and quickens the connecting vessels
>>> Washes away phlegm and opens the portals

Tranquilizes the liver qi
Confluent point of the *shao yang, yang ming,* and
yang wei mai

Dai Mai (GB 26)

Frees the flow of the kidney qi
Subdues counterflow fire of the liver
Stops abnormal vaginal discharge
Clears and disinhibits damp heat
Regulates the menses
Frees the channels and quickens the connecting
vessels

Huan Tiao (GB 30)

Disperses wind dampness in the channels and four
extremities
Disinhibits the low back and knees
Frees the flow of the channels

Yang Ling Quan (GB 34)

Harmonizes the liver
Dries dampness and transforms phlegm
Soothes the sinews
Disinhibits the liver and gallbladder
Fortifies the spleen
Clears gallbladder heat
Clears heat and eliminates dampness
Strengthens the sinews and bones
Hui meeting point of the sinews
He sea point of the foot *shao yang*

Guang Ming (GB 37)

Clears and discharges fire from the liver and
gallbladder
Rectifies the liver

Brightens the eyes and disinhibits vision
Dispels wind and disinhibits dampness
Luo point of the foot *shao yang*

Xuan Zhong (aka *Jue Gu*, GB 39)
Harmonizes the liver
Induces the qi and blood downward
Discharges gallbladder fire
Clears marrow heat (as in steaming bones)
Expels wind and dampness from the channels and
  connecting vessels
Dispels heat of the three foot yang
Confluent point of the three foot yang
Hui meeting point of the marrow

Zu Lin Qi (GB 41)
Out-thrusts and drains the liver and gallbladder
Regulates and rectifies the *dai mai*
Clears fire and extinguishes wind
Brightens the eyes and sharpens hearing
Transforms obstructing phlegm heat
Dispels phlegm and blood stasis from the *jue yin*
Hui meeting point of the *dai mai*
Shu stream point of the foot *shao yang*

Foot *Jue Yin* Liver Channel

Da Dun (Liv 1)
Frees liver wood so as to resolve depressive qi
Warms the liver and the lower sap
Rectifies the lower burner
Harmonizes the *ying* and qi
Returns yang and stems inversion
Regulates menstruation

Treats cold *shan*
Promotes the liver's function of treasuring the
   blood
Jing well point of foot *jue yin*

Xing Jian (Liv 2)

Discharges fire from the liver
Out-thrusts depressive qi
Rectifies the liver qi
Clears the heart and quiets the spirit
Resolves depression
Cools blood heat
Clears the lower burner
Extinguishes wind
Clears heat and drains fire
Courses the channels and quickens the connecting
   vessels
Rong spring point of the foot *jue yin*

Tai Chong (Liv 3)

Frees the flow of liver qi
Descends counterflow qi
Harmonizes the liver
Settles wind
Clears heat from the liver and gallbladder
Stops vomiting
Discharges damp heat in the lower burner
Clears liver fire and subdues liver yang
Rectifies the blood
Opens the channels
Yuan source point of the foot *jue yin*

Qu Quan (Liv 8)

Rectifies the liver

Abducts the turbid downward
Disinhibits the bladder
Drains liver fire
Disinhibits the lower burner
Clears and eliminates dampness and heat
Soothes the sinews
He sea point of the foot *jue yin*

Zhang Men (Liv 13)
Fortifies the spleen
Disperses food stagnation
Relieves fullness and distention
Quickens the blood and transforms stasis
Softens the hard and disperses masses
Rectifies the qi and blood of the viscera and
bowels
Front *mu* point of the spleen
Hui meeting point of the viscera

Qi Men (Liv 14) Removes obstruction from the liver and channels
Quickens the blood and frees the channels
Promotes coursing and discharge of liver qi
Transforms and dispels blood stasis
Dispels evil heat from the blood chamber
Harmonizes the *shao yang fen*
Transforms phlegm
Quiets the liver
Front *mu* point of the liver

Governing Vessel *(Du Mai)*

Chang Qiang (GV 1)
Frees the flow of qi and blood of the anus
Opens the governing and conception vessels

Rectifies the intestines
Harmonizes yin and yang
Disperses swelling and stops pain
Luo point of the governing vessel

Ming Men (GV 4)

Supplements the kidneys and invigorates yang
Nourishes the *yuan* original qi
Disinhibits the lumbus
Secures the essence and stops vaginal discharge
Soothes the sinews and harmonizes the blood

Da Zhui (GV 14)

Disperses yang pathogens so as to out-thrust heat
Diffuses and disinhibits the yang qi
Relieves the exterior and frees the flow of yang
Clears the brain and quiets the spirit
Clears lung heat
Rectifies the qi
Confluent point of all the yang channels

Feng Fu (GV 16)

Dispels wind in general from the body
Expels wind evils in the common cold (*gan mao*)
Clears the essence spirit
Disinhibits the joints
Drains fire

Bai Hui (GV 20)

Opens the sensory portals and resuscitates
Quiets the spirit
Extinguishes liver wind
Upbears clear yang
Clears up-flaming fire in the yang channels

Opens the portals of the upper burner so as to
clear the head and eyes
Confluent point of the three hand and foot yang
channels and the *du mai*

Ren Zhong (GV 26)
Opens the portals and resuscitates
Quiets the spirit
Clears the essence spirit
Clears internal heat
Disinhibits the lumbus
Rectifies counterflow qi of the *yang ming*
Treats wind edema of the face
Dispels wind pathogens

Conception Vessel (*Ren Mai*)

Zhong Ji (CV 3)
Assists the transforming function of the qi *vis à
vis* the bladder
Regulates the blood chamber
Clears and eliminates damp heat
Disinhibits the bladder
Rectifies the lower burner
Warms the essence palace
Front *mu* point of the bladder

Guan Yuan (CV 4)
Warms the lower burner and the uterus
Reinforces the sap
Strengthens the kidney qi
Regulates and supplements the *chong* and *ren*
Warms and regulates the blood chamber and
essence palace

Dispels cold and dampness in the genitals
Separates the clear and turbid
Safeguards health and prevents disease
Strengthens the function of stopping abnormal
  vaginal discharge and restraining the blood
Regulates the qi and invigorates yang
Front *mu* point of the small intestine
Confluent point of the three foot yin and the *ren mai*

Qi Hai (CV 6) Cultivates the sap
Rectifies the qi
Regulates and rectifies the *yuan* source qi of the
  entire body
Promotes the restraint of the blood within its
  channels
Clears and discharges fire from the liver and
  gallbladder
Clears and discharges evil heat from the blood
  division
Supplements the qi
Warms the lower and middle burners
Supplements kidney vacuity
Regulates the menses and stops vaginal discharge
Dispels damp turbidity
Harmonizes the *ying* and blood

Shui Fen (CV 9)
Warms the middle burner
Dispels cold
Promotes diuresis and percolates dampness
Rectifies the bladder qi

Zhong Wan (CV 12)
Rectifies the middle qi

71

Harmonizes the stomach qi
Warms the stomach and intestines
Facilitates upbearing of the clear and downbearing
  of the turbid
Disperses food stagnation
Fortifies the spleen and disinhibits dampness
Front *mu* point of the stomach
Hui meeting point of the bowels

Shang Wan (CV 13)

Clears heat from the heart and stomach
Warms the stomach
Scatters cold
Rectifies the spleen and stomach
Transforms phlegm turbidity
Courses the qi

Ju Que (CV 14)

Removes stagnant fluids from the chest and
  diaphragm
Front *mu* point of the heart
Transforms depressive dampness in the middle
  burner
Clears heat and quiets the spirit
Rectifies the qi and frees the middle

Shan Zhong (CV 17)

Upbears the spleen qi
Downbears stomach qi
Resolves depression
Rectifies and smoothes the circulation of qi in the
  upper burner
Downbears phlegm turbidity
Downbears counterflow lung qi
Clears the lungs and transforms phlegm

Loosens the chest
Front *mu* point of the pericardium
Hui meeting point of the qi

Tian Tu (CV 22)

Frees the flow and rectifies the lung qi
Cools the throat and clears the voice
Stops hiccough and coughing
Diffuses the lungs and transforms phlegm

Functions of Major Two Point Combinations

Lie Que (Lu 7)
+ *Zhao Hai* (Ki 6) Disinhibits the nose and throat
Abducts vacuity fire downward
Nourishes yin
Stops coughing

+ *Fei Shu* (BL 13) Clears heat from the lungs

+ *Chi Ze* (Lu 5) Rectifies the lung qi
Clears heat
Stops coughing
Stops bleeding (hemoptysis)

+ *Tai Yuan* (Lu 9) Strongly diffuses the lung qi and stops
coughing

San Yin Jiao (Sp 6)
+ *Tai Xi* (Ki 3) Nourishes yin
Clears vacuity heat
Stops bleeding (epistaxis due to vacuity heat)

73

Supplements the kidneys

+ *Zhong Ji* (CV 3) Rectifies the qi of the lower burner
Disinhibits urination
Clears heat from the urogenital tract

+ *Xing Jian* (Liv 2) Quickens the blood
Dispels blood stasis

+ *Xue Hai* (Sp 10) Clears heat from the blood division

+ *Da Dun* (Liv 1) Stops abnormal vaginal bleeding

+ *Fu Liu* (Ki 7) Clears heat from the constructive division

+ *Ran Gu* (Ki 2) Supplements the kidneys
Secures the essence

Qi Men (Liv 14)
+ *Ri Yue* (GB 25) Harmonizes the liver
Resolves liver depression

+ *Tai Chong* (Liv 3)
Courses the liver and rectifies the qi
Rectifies the blood
Soothes the liver
Descends counterflow qi
Relieves (abdominal) distention
Stops (abdominal) pain

+ *Xing Jian* (Liv 2) Courses the liver and rectifies the qi

Zu San Li (St 36)
+ *Zhong Wan* (CV 12)

Boosts the stomach qi
Fortifies the spleen
Supplements the qi of the middle burner
Promotes the transportation and
  transformation of the spleen qi
Disperses food stagnation
Upbears the clear and downbears the turbid
Clears the stomach
Transforms phlegm
Harmonizes the stomach qi
Eliminates dampness

+ *Tian Tu* (CV 22) Downbears stomach qi to stop hiccoughing

+ *Shan Zhong* (CV 17)

Descends counterflow qi to stop vomiting

+ *Shang Ju Xu* (St 37)

Disperses food stagnation of the stomach and
  intestines

+ *Zhi Gou* (TH 6) Dispels blood stasis
Rectifies the qi

+ *San Yin Jiao* (Sp 6)

Treats vacuity cold of the spleen and stomach
Supplements the qi and blood
Rectifies the spleen and stomach
Cultivates the root of acquired essence
Supplements the spleen
Nourishes the blood
Descends counterflow qi

+ *Shang Wan* (CV 13)
     Loosens the middle
     Rectifies the middle qi
     Transforms and eliminates phlegm dampness
     Removes accumulation

+ *Jie Xi* (St 41) Eliminates dampness
     Clears heat
     Treats erysipelas of the upper and lower
      extremities

+ *Pi Shu* (Bl 20) Disinhibits the root of postnatal qi and blood
      production
     Supplements the qi and blood
     Banks the qi of the middle burner

+ *Tian Shu* (St 25) Harmonizes the stomach and fortifies the
      spleen
     Opens the bowels and downbears the turbid
     Facilitates the cooperation of earth and water
      in the transportation and transformation of
      grains and liquids
     Opens the bowels
     Stops diarrhea

Nei Guan (Per 6)
+ *Tai Chong* (Liv 3)
     Harmonizes the liver
     Descends counterflow qi

+ *Tai Yuan* (Lu 9) Disinhibits the qi
     Stops wheezing

+ *Zu San Li* (St 36) Rectifies the middle qi

Harmonizes the stomach qi
Stops vomiting

+ *Gong Sun* (Sp 4) Frees the flow of the qi and blood of the
middle burner

+ *Ren Zhong* (GV 26)
Clears heat
Opens the portals
Clears the mind and resuscitates

+ *San Yin Jiao* (Sp 6)
Nourishes yin
Clears fire
Disinhibits the qi
Nourishes the heart to quicken the blood
Supplements the heart to nourish blood

+ *Li Dui* (St 45) Discharges stomach fire

+ *Qu Chi* (Li 11) Loosens the chest
Clears heat

+ *Zhong Wan* (CV 12)
Harmonizes the middle burner
Loosens the chest
Descends counterflow stomach qi

+ *Shan Zhong* (CV 17)
Loosens the chest
Resolves depression
Soothes the qi
Descends counterflow qi
Stops coughing due to stagnation of chest
qi

+ *Jian Li* (CV 11)   Opens the portals of the chest and diaphragm
Harmonizes the stomach to stop vomiting
Opens the portals of the chest to resolve
   depression
Discharges heart fire
Quiets the spirit

Zhong Wan (CV 12)
+ *Feng Long* (St 40)

> Rectifies the channel qi of the spleen and
>   stomach
> Transforms and eliminates phlegm dampness

+ *Xing Jian* (Liv 2) Resolves depression
Loosens the middle

+ *Tian Shu* (St 25) Rectifies the qi of the stomach and intestines
Disperses food stagnation
Downbears turbidity

+ *Zhang Men* (Liv 13)

> Regulates and rectifies the function of the
> spleen and stomach to eliminate phlegm
> dampness

+ *Qi Hai* (CV 6)   Warms the middle burner and scatters cold
   to stop diarrhea
Dispels cold and eliminates dampness
Warms the middle and rectifies the qi

+ *Jian Shi* (Per 5) Resolves depression
Loosens the chest

+ *Pi Shu* (Bl 20)   Rectifies and regulates the function of the
                     spleen and stomach
                     Eliminates dampness

Yang Ling Quan (GB 34)
+ *Shui Fen* (CV 9)   Abducts water downward
                     Disinhibits urination and, therefore, also
                     bowel movements

+ *Jia Xi* (GB 43)   Clears and eliminates damp heat of the liver
                     and gallbladder

+ *Zhong Wan* (CV 12)
                     Fortifies the spleen and stomach *vis à vis*
                     transportation and transformation

+ *Xing Jian* (Liv 2) Harmonizes the liver
                     Resolves depression
                     Course the liver and rectifies the qi
                     Clears heat from the liver and gallbladder

+ *Gong Sun* (Sp 4) Fortifies the spleen
                     Eliminates dampness

+ *Tai Chong* (Liv 3)
                     Harmonizes the liver
                     Stops pain
                     Subdues counterflow liver wood qi
                     Frees the flow of the channel qi of the liver
                     and gallbladder

+ *San Yin Jiao* (Sp 6)
                     Clears and eliminates damp heat from the
                     stomach and intestines

Fortifies the spleen
Eliminates dampness

+ *Qu Chi* (Li 11) Frees the flow of the channels
Disinhibits the sinews and bones
Diffuses the qi
Downbears turbidity
Discharges fire
Removes obstruction of the sinews
Disinhibits the joints
Treats *bi zheng* (obstruction patterns)

+ *Xue Hai* (Sp 10) Clears heat from the blood division
Fortifies the spleen
Regulates the menses

+ *Zhi Gou* (TH 6) Frees the flow of the qi and quickens the
blood to treat hypochondriac pain
Dispels blood stasis

+ *Huan Tiao* (GB 30)
Removes obstruction from the channels
Disperses exterior pathogenic factors
Rectifies the qi and blood
Expels wind
Eliminates dampness

+ *Pi Shu* (Bl 20) Transforms dampness
Clears heat
Fortifies the spleen and clears and eliminates
damp heat

+ *Xuan Zhong* (aka *Jue Gu*, GB 39)
Strengthens the sinews and bones
Treats *wei zheng* (atony patterns)

He Gu (Li 4)

+ *Tai Chong* (Li 3) Opens the portals
Subdues liver yang
Rectifies the qi and blood
Removes obstruction from the channels

+ *Qu Chi* (Li 11) Clears heat
Expels wind
Dispels wind and clears heat and disinhibits
the stomach and intestines to out-thrust
rashes

+ *Tai Yuan* (Lu 9) Promotes the lungs' diffusion and depurative
downbearing

+ *Lie Que* (Lu 7) Treats edema in the upper body
Relieves the exterior

+ *Da Ling* (Per 7) Clears fire from the middle burner
Resolves depression
Quiets the spirit

+ *Fei Shu* (Bl 13) Clears heat from the upper burner to protect
lung yin

+ *Fu Liu* (Ki 7) Regulates diaphoresis

+ *Ying Xiang* (LI 20)
Clears wind heat from the *yang ming*
Removes obstruction from the portals of the
nose

+ *Nei Ting* (St 44) Discharges *yang ming* stomach heat
Drains and discharges stomach heat

Discharges the *yang ming* qi in order to clear
heat from the eyes

+ *Jian Shi* (Per 5)   Frees the flow of qi
Resolves depression

Da Zhui (GV 14)
+ *Xian Gu* (St 43)   Drains external evil heat, especially from the
yang ming

+ *Qu Chi* (Li 11)   Expels wind
Clears heat

+ *Wai Guan* (TH 5)
Boosts yang to remove obstruction from the
exterior so as to relieve pain of the head and
body

+ *Feng Chi* (GB 20)
Dispels wind dampness
Clears heat

Xin Shu (Bl 15)
+ *Shen Men* (Ht 7)   Quiets the heart spirit
Opens the portals of the heart
Treats insomnia due to heart and spleen dual
vacuity

+ *Lao Gong* (Per 8)
Subdues heart fire
Quiet the spirit

+ *Ju Que* (CV 14)   Frees the flow of the heart qi in chest *bi*

Drains fire
Quiets the spirit

Shen Shu (Bl 23)
+ *Tai Xi* (Ki 3)   Enriches water so as to control fire
Supplements the kidneys
Fulfills the essence

+ *Ming Men* (GV 4)
Supplements the kidneys
Invigorates yang

+ *Guan Yuan* (CV 4)
Supplements the kidneys
Treats kidney vacuity diarrhea

+ *San Yin Jiao* (Sp 6)
Supplements the kidneys
Enriches yin

Qu Chi (Li 11)
+ *San Yin Jiao* (Sp 6)
Clears heat from the blood
Extinguishes liver wood wind
Frees the channels and dispels blood stasis

+ *He Gu* (Li 4)   Clears heat from the upper burner

+ *Zhi Gou* (TH 6)   Clears heat
Treats skin lesions (such as *she chuan chuang,*
cluster of snakes sores, *i.e.,* herpes zoster

+ *Jian Yu* (Li 15)   Rectifies lung qi

                    Quickens the blood
                    Extinguishes wind and dispels evil qi (from
                        the channels)

+ *Nei Ting* (St 44) Clears and downbears the turbid so as to clear
                        the stomach and intestines
                    Clears and discharges evil heat from the
                        stomach and intestines
                    Clears pathogenic heat from the *yang ming*
                    Clears accumulated heat from the *yang ming*

+ *Xian Gu* (St 43) Clears evil heat from the *yang ming*

Yu Ji (Lu 10)
+ *Shao Shang* (Lu 11)
                    Drains lung fire to stop sore throat

+ *Shao Ze* (SI 1)   Disinhibits the breast
                    Promotes lactation

+ *Chi Ze* (Lu 5)   Clears heat from the lungs

Guan Yuan (CV 4)
+ *Bai Hui* (GV 20) Secures the qi
                    Raises yang
                    Resuscitates

+ *Shen Shu* (Bl 23) Invigorates the source of fire
                    Invigorates yang qi
                    Dispels cold and dampness

+ *Tai Xi* (Ki 3)   Supplements kidney yang
                    Treats diarrhea due to kidney vacuity

84

Xing Jian (Liv 2)
+ *Feng Chi* (GB 20)
>> Clears the head
>> Drains liver fire

+ *Yong Quan* (Ki 1)
>> Nourishes yin
>> Harmonizes the liver

+ *Zhong Ji* (CV 3) Clears liver fire from the lower burner

+ *Zu Lin Qi* (GB 41)
>> Clears fire from the liver and gallbladder

Zhang Men (Liv 13)
+ *Nei Ting* (St 44) Disperses food stagnation
>> Relieves abdominal distention

+ *Pi Shu* (Bl 20) Warms cold and eliminates dampness
>> Recedes yin jaundice

Feng Long (St 40)
+ *Nei Ting* (St 44) Frees the flow of bowel qi

+ *Tian Tu* (CV 22) Soothes the qi
>> Transforms phlegm

Ren Zhong (GV 26)
+ *Yin Tang* (extra point)
>> Resuscitates the mind
>> Opens clenched teeth (as in epilepsy and
>> tetanus)

+ *Bai Hui* (GV 20) Regulates and rectifies the yang qi of the *du mai* and hand three yang

Opens the portals and arouses the brain

Xuan Zhong (aka *Jue Gu*, GB 39)
+ *Da Shu* (Bl 11) Strengthens the sinews and builds the bone

+ *Zhong Feng* (Liv 4)

Drains the liver and supplements the spleen

Jia Che (St 6)
+ *Yi Feng* (TH 17) Frees the flow of the channels

Relieves difficulty in chewing

+ *Xia Guan* (St 7) Relieves clenched teeth

Guan Chong (TH 1)
+ *Shao Shang* (Lu 11)

Disperses hidden evils from the viscera and bowels

Clears heat and resolves toxins

+ *Shang Yang* (LI 1)

Clears heat from the three burners

Clears heat from the stomach

Shen Men (Ht 7)
+ *Jian Shi* (Per 5) Frees the flow of the heart and pericardium channels

Opens the portals of the heart

Arouses the brain (*i.e.*, resuscitates)

+ *Xi Men* (Per 4)   Tranquilizes the source of heart yang
Treats palpitations

Bai Hui (GV 20)
+ *Xi Men* (Per 4)   Regulates and rectifies the yang qi of the *du mai*
Assists the qi's function of restraining the blood of the *chong* and *ren*

Lao Gong (Per 8)
+ *Da Ling* (Per 7)   Clears heat from the pericardium
Clears fire from the heart

Lian Quan (CV 23)
+ *Tian Tu* (CV 22)   Descends counterflow qi
Disinhibits the throat

Tian Shu (St 25)
+ *Gui Lai* (St 29)   Clears heat (from the lower burner)
Regulates the menses

+ *Liang Men* (St 21)
Disperses food stagnation

Xue Hai (Sp 10)
+ *Shui Quan* (Ki 5)   Clears heat from the blood
Stops bleeding

Shan Zhong (CV 17)
+ *Shao Ze* (SI 1)   Rectifies the qi

Promotes lactation

+ *Fei Shu* (Bl 13) Rectifies the lungs
Soothes the chest qi *(zong qi)*

Pang Guang Shu (Bl 28)
+ *Zhong Ji* (CV 3) Clears and eliminates damp heat from the
bladder
Disinhibits urination

+ *Xiao Chang Shu* (Bl 27)
Disinhibits urination
Clears summerheat

Tai Yuan (Lu 9)
+ *Fu Liu* (Ki 7) Restores the pulse in emergency situations
Raises clear yang

+ *Chi Ze* (Lu 5) Clears heat
Frees the flow of qi
Stops coughing
Stops wheezing

Wei Shu (Bl 20)
+ *San Yin Jiao* (Bl 22)
Treats external pathogens invading the
stomach and intestines

Jin Jin *(extra point)*
+ *Yu Ye* (extra point) Prevents outflow of fluids (*i.e.*, oral dribbling)
Stops thirst and engenders fluids

Clears heat
Relieves vexation

Da Heng (Sp 15)   Opens the bowels
+ *Da Chang Shu* (Bl 25)

Chang Qiang (GV 1)
+ *Cheng Shan* (Bl 57)
                    Clears and eliminates damp heat from the
                        large intestine
                    Treats the blood (as in hemorrhoids)

Xiao Chang Shu (Bl 27)
+ *Xia Ju Xu* (St 39) Clears and opens the bowels

Wei Shu (Bl 21)
+ *Pi Shu* (Bl 20)   Rectifies the middle qi
                  Supplements the middle (burner)
                  Benefits the root of acquired qi and blood

Shen Que (CV 8)   Dispels cold
+ *Qi Hai* (CV 6)   Stems yang desertion
                  Resolves depression
                  Warms the middle burner

Gan Shu (Bl 18)
+ *Ge Shu* (Bl 17)   Nourishes the blood
                  Harmonizes the liver
                  Quickens the blood and dispels stasis

+ *Tai Chong* (Liv 3)
　　　　　　　　Resolves depression

Tian Zhu (Bl 10)
+ *Yi Feng* (TH 17)　Clears the mind
　　　　　　　　Drains liver fire

Shui Fen (CV 9)
+ *Jian Li* (CV 11)　Regulates water (metabolism)
　　　　　　　　Disinhibits urination

Zhong Ji (CV 13)　Stops pain
+ *Da Ju* (St 27)　Dispels blood stasis

Jian Jing (GB 21)
+ *Ru Gen* (St 18)　Rectifies the qi
　　　　　　　　Disperses swelling (of the breasts)

Er Men (TH 21)
+ *Ting Hui* (GB 2)　Frees the flow of qi locally
　　　　　　　　Opens the portals (of the ear)
　　　　　　　　Disinhibits hearing

Fei Shu (Bl 13)
+ *Feng Men* (Bl 12)
　　　　　　　　Dispels external evils from the exterior
　　　　　　　　Loosens the chest
　　　　　　　　Rectifies the lung qi

Shen Mai (Bl 62)
+ *Kun Lun* (Bl 60) Removes obstruction from the *tai yang*
                    Treats stiff neck and upper and lower back

Dai Mai (GB 26)
+ *Wu Shu* (GB 27) Stops abnormal vaginal discharge

Ying Xiang (LI 20)
+ *Yin Tang* (extra point)
                    Clears fire (locally)
                    Disinhibits the nose

Shen Zhu (GV 12) Drains evil yang
+ *Ling Tai* (GV 10) Clears and resolves fire toxins (as in lung
                    abscess)

Functions of Major Three Point Combinations

San Yin Jiao (Sp 6)
+ *Shen Men* (Ht 7) Nourishes the blood
+ *Ju Que* (CV 14) Quiets the spirit

+ *Zu San Li* (St 36) Fortifies the spleen
+ *Pi Shu* (Bl 20)   Benefits the root of postnatal qi and blood
                    production

+ *Zu San Li* (St 36) Supplements the spleen
+ *Zhong Wan* (CV 12)
                    Rectifies the qi and controls the blood

+ *Zu San Li* (St 36) Fortifies the spleen
+ *Shen Men* (Ht 7) Rectifies the qi
                         Controls the blood
                         Quiets the spirit

+ *Fu Liu* (Ki 7) Nourishes yin
+ *Zhao Hai* (Ki 6) Moistens dryness

+ *Shen Shu* (Bl 23) Supplements the kidneys
+ *Ran Gu* (Ki 2) Nourishes yin

+ *Shen Shu* (Bl 23) Supplements the kidneys
+ *Da Heng* (Ki 12) Secures the essence
                         Treats spermatorrhea without dreams

+ *Shen Shu* (Bl 23) Supplements the kidneys
+ *Tai Xi* (Ki 3) Nourishes yin

+ *Shen Shu* (Bl 23) Harmonizes the spleen and stomach
+ *Gong Sun* (Sp 4) Eliminates dampness

+ *Qi Hai* (CV 6) Supplements the spleen
+ *Zhong Wan* (CV 12)
                         Supplements the qi and blood

+ *Qi Hai* (CV 6) Frees the flow of qi and dispels blood stasis
+ *Guan Yuan* (CV 4)
                         Supplements the qi
                         Nourishes the blood

+ *Xue Hai* (Sp 10) Frees the flow of qi
+ *Xing Jian* (Liv 2) Quickens the blood

+ *Nei Guan* (Per 6) Relieves vexation
+ *Xue Hai* (Sp 10) Quiets the spirit

Tai Chong (Liv 3)
+ *Zu Lin Qi* (GB 41)
+ *Qiu Xu* (GB 40) Resolves depression
                    Discharges liver fire

+ *Gan Shu* (Bl 18) Clears fire from the liver and gallbladder
+ *Dan Shu* (Bl 19) Clears fire and eases the mind

+ *Yang Ling Quan* (GB 34)
+ *Qu Chi* (Li 11) Harmonizes the liver
                    Relieves convulsions and contractions of the
                        four extremities

+ *Yang Ling Quan* (GB 34)
+ *Xing Jian* (Liv 2) Harmonizes the liver
                      Resolves depression

Zu San Li (St 36)
+ *Zhong Wan* (CV 12)
+ *Feng Long* (St 40)
                    Clears internal heat
                    Transforms stubborn or old phlegm

+ *Zhong Wan* (CV 12)
+ *Tian Shu* (Bl 25) Precipitate stagnant heat
                     Harmonizes the middle burner
                     Stops vomiting

+ *Zhong Wan* (CV 12)
+ *Pi Shu* (Bl 20) Fortifies the spleen
                    Harmonizes the stomach
                    Eliminates dampness
                    Transforms phlegm

+ *Zhong Wan* (CV 12)

+ *Tian Tu* (CV 22) Rectifies the qi
                           Descends counterflow qi
                           Stops vomiting

+ *Zhi Gou* (TH 6) Promotes bowel movements
+ *Da Chang Shu* (Bl 25)

+ *Tian Shu* (St 25) Abducts the qi downward
+ *Gui Lai* (St 29)   Rectifies the spleen and stomach

He Gu (Li 4)
+ *Tai Chong* (Liv 3) Stops pain and convulsions
+ *Shen Zhu* (GV 12) Treats opisthotonos

+ *Shang Ju Xu* (St 37)
+ *Xia Ju Xu* (St 39) Clears accumulation of heat from the
                                intestines

+ *Nei Ting* (St 44) Clears damp heat from the stomach and
+ *Yang Ling Quan*   intestines
  (GB 34)   Treats damp heat diarrhea

+ *Wai Guan* (TH 5) Dispels external evils from the exterior
+ *Da Zhui* (GV 14) Recedes fever

+ *Feng Chi* (GB 20) Expels wind
+ *Jing Ming* (Bl 1) Clears heat (from the eyes causing red eyes
                           and eye pain)

+ *Gan Shu* (Bl 18) Extinguishes wind
+ *Jian Shi* (Per 5) Resolves depression
                           Treats emotional depression and qi stagnation

Guan Yuan (CV 4)
+ *Shen Que* (CV 8) Abducts yang to its lower source
+ *Bai Hui* (GV 20) Rescues from dying

+ *Zhong Ji* (CV 3) Supplements the *chong* and *ren*
+ *Dai Mai* (GB 26) Supplements the *zong* or chest qi

+ *Zhong Ji* (CV3) Supplements vacuity detriment of the lower
+ *Qi Hai* (CV 6)   burner

+ *Qi Hai* (CV 6)   Abducts yang to its lower source
+ *Shen Qui* (CV 8) Stems desertion

+ *Xia Ju Xu* (St 39) Clears heat from the intestines
+ *Xiao Chang Shu* (Bl 27)
                   Treats bloody dysentery
                   Abducts stagnation downward

+ *Tian Shu* (St 25) Scatters cold
+ *Zhong Wan* (CV 12)
                   Warms the stomach and intestines

+ *Zu San Li* (St 36) Boosts the *yuan* original qi
+ *Qi Hai* (CV 6)

Yang Ling Quan (GB 34)
+ *Xuan Zhong* (aka *Jue Gu*, GB 39)
+ *Da Shu* (Bl 11) Strengthens the sinews and bones

+ *Huan Tiao* (GB 30)
+ *Yin Ling Quan* (Sp 9)
                   Scatters cold
                   Dispels wind

Eliminates dampness
Frees the flow of the channels

Tian Shu (St 25)
+ *Liang Men* (St 21) Descends stomach qi counterflow
+ *Zhong Wan* (CV 12)

+ *Shang Ju Xu* (St 37)
+ *Qu Chi* (LI 11)   Eliminates accumulation from the intestines
                     Clears and eliminates damp heat
                     Stops pain (as is appendicitis or intestinal
                        abscess)

Shen Shu (Bl 23)
+ *Fu Liu* (Ki 7)   Supplements the kidneys to aid their grasping
+ *Tai Xi* (Ki 3)   the qi

Wei Shu (Bl 21)
+ *Zhong Wan* (CV 12)
+ *Pi Shu* (Bl 20)   Scatters cold
                     Eliminates dampness
                     Treats yin jaundice
                     Warms the middle burner
Wei Zhong (Bl 40)
+ *Xue Hai* (Sp 10) Resolves damp toxins
+ *Ge Shu* (Bl 17)   Clears heat from the blood
                     Treats skin diseases

Feng Chi (GB 20)
+ *Ren Zhong* (GV 26)
+ *Ying Xiang* (LI 20)
                     Stops pain
                     Dispel wind and eliminate dampness

Bai Hui (GV 20)
+ *Yin Tang* (extra point)
+ *Ren Zhong* (GV 26)

      Arouses the mind
      Opens the portals

Zhong Wan (CV 12)
+ *Pi Shu* (Bl 20) Rectifies the middle qi
+ *Feng Long* (St 40)

      Transforms phlegm

Zan Zhu (Bl 2)
+ *Jing Ming* (Bl 1) Clears heat
+ *Zu Lin Qi* (GB 41)

      Brightens the eyes

Guan Chong (TH 1)
+ *Shao Shang* (Lu 11)
+ *Chi Ze* (Lu 5) Opens the portals (in heat stroke)

      Drains summerheat

5

Choosing Points Based on Principle (2)

(Translated from *Zhong Guo Zhen Jiu Chu Fang Xue [The Theory of Prescription Writing in Chinese Acupuncture/Moxibustion]* by Xiao Shao-qing)[19]

To start sweating: *He Gu* (LI 4), *Fu Liu* (Ki 7), & *Da Shu* (Bl 11). (This combination) mainly treats fever without sweating due to external invasion.

To stop sweating: *Yin Xi* (Ht 6), *Hou Xi* (SI 3), *He Gu* (LI 4). Mainly treats night sweats and spontaneous perspiration.

To stop vomiting: *Nei Guan* (Per 6), *Zu San Li* (St 36), *Zhong Wan* (CV 12), *Gong Sun* (Sp 4), *Zhong Kui* (Middle Chief, extra point, located at the medial end of the distal phalangeal joint of the third finger), *Shan Zhong* (CV 17), and *Lao Gong* (Per 8). Mainly treats vomiting, hiccup, and acid regurgitation.

To initiate vomiting: *Nei Guan* (Per 6) and *Zhong Wan* (CV 12). Mainly treats food accumulation and nausea with a desire to vomit. Commonly, injury due to digestive disorder will lead to nausea with a desire to vomit. Needle *Nei Guan* and strongly drain *Zhong Wan*.

To promote bowel movements: *Tian Shu* (St 25), *Da Chang Shu*

---

[19] Xiao Shao-qing, *op. cit.*

(Bl 25), *Zu San Li* (St 36), *Feng Long* (St 40), *Zhi Gou* (TH 6), *Yang Ling Quan* (GB 34), and *Da Dun* (Liv 1). Mainly treats constipation due to the bowels not freely flowing.

To stop diarrhea: *Tian Shu* (St 25), *Da Chang Shu* (Bl 25), *Zu San Li* (St 36), *Da Heng* (Sp 15), *Si Yu Shi Zi* (Four Corners/Ten Writings, *i.e.*, *Liang Men* [St 21], *Da Ju* [St 27], *Shui Fen* [CV 9], *Shen Que* [CV 8], *Qi Hai* [CV 6], *Tian Shu* [St 25]); moxa. Mainly treats watery feces and loose diarrhea, including spleen vacuity diarrhea and kidney vacuity diarrhea.

To disperse food stagnation: *Zu San Li* (St 36), *Gong Sun* (Sp 4), *Pi Shu* (Bl 20), and *Xuan Ji* (CV 21). Mainly treats poor digestion and food stagnation.

To eliminate and disperse (accumulations, *i.e.*, lumps or masses): *Tian Jing* (TH 10) and *Shao Hai* (Ht 3); moxa 7 cones. *Zhou Jian* (tip of the olecranon process), *Bai Lao* (extra point, located 1 *cun* lateral to C5), and *A Shi* (points where painful). (This first combination) mainly treats swollen nodes (in the neck). *He Gu* (LI 4), *Shao Shang* (Lu 11), *Que Shang* (extra point, location unknown), and *Zhao Hai* (Ki 6). (This second combination) mainly treats breast moth (*i.e.*, mastitis).

To harmonize and dispel: *Tao Dao* (GV 13), *Jian Shi* (Per 5), *Wai Guan* (TH 5), and *Hou Xi* (SI 3). Mainly treats *nue* (malaria) and alternating fever and chills.

To clear heat: *Da Zhui* (GV 14), *He Gu* (LI 4), *Qu Chi* (LI 11), *Tao Dao* (GV 13), *Xian Gu* (St 43), and *Nei Ting* (St 44). Mainly treats all sorts of hot diseases, including externally contracted malaria.

To warm the middle and stem yang (desertion): Moxa *Qi Hai*

(CV 6), *Guan Yuan* (CV 4), and *Shen Que* (CV 8; indirect moxa on top of salt). Needle and moxa *Zu San Li* (St 36), *Nei Guan* (Per 6), and *Bai Hui* (GV 20). Mainly treats facial pallor, cold limbs, excessive perspiration, and a minute pulse about to disappear, for example, stroke, desertion patterns, etc.

To supplement the qi: *Qi Hai* (CV 6), *Guan Yuan* (CV 4), *Zhong Wan* (CV 12), and *Zu San Li* (St 36). Mainly treats insufficiency of middle qi and qi vacuity and fall patterns, as in stomach ptosis, etc.

To supplement the blood: *Pi Shu* (Bl 20), *Zhang Men* (Liv 13), *Ge Shu* (Bl 17), and *San Yin Jiao* (Sp 6). Mainly treats blood vacuity, loss of blood, *beng lou*[20], and other such patterns.

To invigorate yang: *Ming Men* (GV 4), *Shen Shu* (Bl 23), *Jing Gong* (Bl 52), *Guan Yuan* (CV 4), *Qi Hai* (CV 6), and *Guan Yuan Shu* (Bl 26). Mainly treats atonic yang (impotence), nocturnal emission, and seminal incontinence.

To stop cough: *Lie Que* (Lu 7), *Tai Yuan* (Lu 9), *Chi Ze* (Lu 5), and *Fei Shu* (Bl 13). Mainly treats cough and stuffy chest.

To stabilize wheezing: *Lie Que* (Lu 7), *Si Feng* (extra points, the four proximal interphalangeal points), *Ding Chuan* (extra point), *Chuan Xi* (extra point), and *Shan Zhong* (CV 17). Mainly treats shallow wheezing.

To transform phlegm: *Feng Long* (St 40), *Zhong Wan* (CV 12), *Nei Guan* (Per 6), *Ju Que* (CV 14), and *Pi Shu* (Bl 20). Mainly

---

[20] *Beng lou* is usually translated as uterine bleeding. This is, in Chinese, a compound term in which *beng* means profuse hemorrhagic bleeding and *lou* means continuous metrorrhagic trickle.

treats chest and epigastric distention with excessive, suffocating phlegm.

To rectify the qi: *Shan Zhong* (CV 17), *Qi Hai* (CV 6), and *Ge Shu* (Bl 17). Mainly treats stuffy chest due to qi counterflow, borborygmus due to qi stagnation, and such patterns.

To arouse the brain: *Ren Zhong* (GV 26) and *Shi Xuan* (extra points). Mainly treats high fever and loss of consciousness.

To tranquilize one's composure: *Bai Hui* (GV 20), *Ding Shen* (Stabilize the Spirit, extra point, located below *Ren Zhong* [GV 26]), *Si Shen Cong* (Four Immortals, extra points), *Yao Qi* (extra point below the spinous process of S2), *Jian Shi* (Per 5), *Hou Xi* (SI 3), *Feng Long* (St 40), and *Yong Quan* (Ki 1). Mainly treats mania and withdrawal patterns.

To quiet the spirit: *Bai Hui* (GV 20), *Shen Men* (Ht 7), *Nei Guan* (Per 6), *Xin Shu* (Bl 15), *San Yin Jiao* (Sp 6), and *Tai Xi* (Ki 3). Mainly treats loss of sleep, forgetfulness, palpitations, and dream-disturbed sleep.

To relieve spasms: *Bai Hui* (GV 20), *Hou Xi* (SI 3), *Qu Chi* (LI 11), *Yang Ling Quan* (GB 34), *Cheng Shan* (Bl 57), *Tai Chong* (Liv 3), *Kun Lun* (Bl 60), and *Jin Suo* (GV 8). Mainly treats opisthotonos and spasms of the four limbs.

To open the portals and utter sound: *Ya Men* (GV 15), *Liang Quan* (CV 23), *Jia Che* (St 6), *Tong Li* (Ht 5), and *Tian Tu* (CV 22). Mainly treats apoplexy, aphasia, and sudden loss of voice.

To free the vessels: *Nei Guan* (Per 6), *Shen Men* (Ht 7), *Xin Shu* (Bl 15), *Jue Yin Shu* (Bl 14), and *Zu San Li* (St 36). Mainly treats weak pulse conditions, pulseless patterns, and heart failure patterns.

To dispel wind: *Feng Chi* (GB 20), *Feng Fu* (GV 16), *Bai Hui* (GV 20), *Qu Chi* (LI 11), and *Kun Lun* (Bl 60). Mainly treats liver wind, wind damage, headache, and other such conditions.

To disinhibit urination: *Zhong Ji* (CV 3), *Pang Guang Shu* (Bl 28), *San Jiao Shu* (Bl 22), *Yin Ling Quan* (Sp 9), *San Yin Jiao* (Sp 6), *Guan Yuan* (CV 4), and *Shen Shu* (Bl 23). Mainly treats retention of urine and also enuresis, urinary incontinence, etc.

To stop bleeding: *Shang Xing* (GV 23) and *Xue Jian Chou* (extra point between GV 22 and 23). (This first combination) mainly treats epistaxis. *Yu Ji* (Lu 10) and *Chi Ze* (Lu 5). (This second combination) mainly treats cough and hemoptysis. *San Yin Jiao* (Sp 6), *Tai Chong* (Liv 3), and *Yin Bai* (Sp 1). (This combination) treats *beng luo*. *Cheng Shan* (Bl 57), *Kong Zui* (Lu 6), and *Er Bai* (Two Whites, extra point, located between Per 4 and 5). (This combination) treats hemorrhoidal bleeding. For all hemorrhagic conditions, needle *Ge Shu* (Bl 17).

To scatter stagnation: Bleed *Wei Zhong* (Bl 40) to treat acute lumbar strain. Needle *Zu San Li* (St 36) to treat blood stasis in side the chest and mammary abscess. Needle *Da Bao* (Sp 21) and *Yang Ling Quan* (GB 34) to treat injury of the ribs. Needle *Zhong Guan* (extra point, located between Per 7 and 8) and *Da Ling* (Per 7) to treat injury of the wrist joint. Needle *Jian Jing* (GB 21) and *Qu Chi* (LI 11) to treat injury of the shoulder and arm. Needle *Du Bi* (St 35), *Kuan Gu* (Hip Bone, extra point), and *Yang Ling Quan* (GB 34) to treat injury of the knee. Needle *Qiu Xu* (GB 40) and *Kun Lun* (Bl 60) to treat injury of the ankle.

To resolve toxins: *Ling Tai* (GV 10), *He Gu* (LI 4), *Wei Zhong* (Bl 40), *Bai Lao* (extra point, located 1 *cun* below and lateral to CV 5), and *Huan Men* (extra point, location unknown). Mainly treats all types of furuncles, boils, or sores. Use in their initial stage of development.

To produce saliva and quench thirst: *Jin Jin* and *Yu Ye* (extra points), *Zhao Hai* (Ki 6), *San Yin Jiao* (Sp 6), *Ran Gu* (Ki 2), *Tai Xi* (Ki 3), and *Wei Guan Xia Shu* (extra point, located 1 *cun* lateral to T8). Mainly treats dry mouth and thirst (as in thirsting and wasting disease), dry throat.

Dispel wind and soothe the sinews: On the upper limbs, select *Jian Yu* (LI 15), *Qu Chi* (LI 11), *He Gu* (LI 4), and *Jing Bi* (extra point, location unknown). On the lower limbs, select *Huan Tiao* (GB 30) and *Yang Ling Quan* (GB 34) or *Xia Ju Xu* (St 39) and *Jue Gu/Xuan Zhong* (GB 39). Mainly treats stroke, hemiplegia, osteoarthritis, infantile paralysis, etc.

To raise the blood pressure: *Nei Guan* (Per 6) and *Huan Men* (extra point, location unknown). Mainly treats low blood pressure, heart failure, and exhaustion patterns.

To lower the blood pressure: *Yin Ling Quan* (Sp 9), *Zu San Li* (St 36), *Qu Chi* (LI 11) through to *Shao Hai* (Ht 3), and *Tai Chong* (Liv 3) through to *Yong Quan* (Ki 1). Mainly treats high blood pressure.

To open menstruation: *Tian Shu* (St 25), *Shui Dao* (St 28), *Gui Lai* (St 29), *Xue Hai* (Sp 10), *Di Ji* (Sp 8), and *Tai Chong* (Liv 3). Mainly treats irregular menstruation and amenorrhea.

To hasten delivery: *He Gu* (LI 4), *San Yin Jiao* (Sp 6), *Zhi Yin* (Bl 67), *Du Yin* (extra point, located in the center of the metatarso-phalangeal joint crease on the plantar surface of the second toe), and *Kun Lun* (Bl 60). Mainly treats delayed delivery, retained placenta, and sluggish delivery.

To stop pain: *Tai Yang* (extra point), *Feng Chi* (GB 20), *Yin Tang* (extra point), and *He Gu* (LI 4) treat head pain. *Jia Che* (St 6), *Xia Guan* (St 7), *He Gu* (LI 4), and *Nei Ting* (St 44) treat tooth pain. *Shao Shang* (Lu 11), *He Gu* (LI 4), *Que Pen* (St 12), *Tian Tu* (CV 22), and *Zhao Hai* (Ki 6) treat throat pain. *Lie Que* (Lu 7), *Hou Xi* (SI 3), *Tian Zhu* (Bl 10), *Da Zhui* (GV 14), *Luo Zhen* (extra point), and *Kun Lun* (Bl 60) treat back of the neck pain and wry neck. *Nei Guan* (Per 6), *Xi Men* (Per 4), *Shan Zhong* (CV 17), and *Feng Long* (St 40) treat chest pain. *Da Ling* (Per 7), *Shen Men* (Ht 7), *Xi Men* (Per 4), *Xin Shu* (Bl 15), and *Ju Gu* (LI 16) treat angina pectoris. *Zhong Wan* (CV 12), *Nei Guan* (Per 6), *Zu San Li* (St 36), *Nei Ting* (St 44), *Inner Nei Ting* (extra point, located on the plantar surface directly under St 44), and *Gong Sun* (Sp 4) treat stomach pain. *Zhong Wan* (CV 12), *Zu San Li* (St 36), and *San Yin Jiao* (Sp 6) treat abdominal pain. If there is also vomiting, add *Nei Guan* (Per 6). For diarrhea, add *Tian Shu* (St 25). For appendicitis, add *Lan Wei Xue* (extra point) and *Tian Shu* (St 25). If there is painful menstruation, add *Di Ji* (Sp 8) and *Xue Hai* (Sp 10). *Zhi Gou* (TH 6), *Qi Men* (Liv 14), *Ri Yue* (GB 24), *Tai Chong* (Liv 3), *Yang Ling Quan* (GB 34), and *Qiu Xu* (GB 40) mainly treat upper rib pain (due to any liver/gallbladder disease). *Hou Xi* (SI 3), *Ge Shu* (Bl 17), *Ming Men* (GV 4), *Shen Shu* (Bl 23), *Wei Zhong* (Bl 40), and *Kun Lun* (Bl 60) mainly treat lumbar and back pain. *Shi Qi Zhui Xia* (extra point, located below the spinous process of L5), *Ci Liao* (Bl 32), and *Zhi Bian* (Bl 54) mainly treat low back and buttock pain (sacroiliac joint pain), leg pain, and paralysis of the lower limbs. *He Gu* (LI 4), *Hou Xi* (SI 3), and *Ba Xie* (extra points) mainly treat swelling, pain, and numbness of the hand and fingers. *Qu Chi* (LI 11), *Shou San Li* (LI 10), *Tian Jing* (TH 10),and *Shao Hai* (Ht 3) mainly treat elbow joint pain. *Yang Xi* (LI 5), *Zhong Xuan* (extra point, located half way between LI 5 and TH 4), and *Yang Gu* (TH 4) mainly treat wrist joint pain. *Jian Yu* (LI 15), *Jian Liao* (TH 14), *Nao Shu* (SI 10), *Jian Nei Ling* (extra point), and *Ju Gu* (LI 16) mainly treats shoulder joint pain. *Xi Yan* (St 35), *He Ding* (extra point, located above the kneecap), *Xi Zhong* (extra point, location unknown), *Kuan Gu* (extra point, located 1.5 *cun* to the left and right of St 34), *Yang Ling Quan* (GB 34), *Xi Shang* (extra point, located 4.5 *cun* above the patella), and *Er Xue* (extra point, location unknown) mainly treat knee joint pain. *Huan Tiao* (GB 30), *Cheng Fu* (Bl 36), *Huan Zhong* (extra point, located in the center of the gluteus), *Zhi Bian* (Bl 54), and *Jue Gu* (GB 39) mainly treat hip joint pain and sciatica. *Bi Guan* (St 31), *Fu Tu* (St 32), *Si Qiang* (extra point, located 4 *cun* above the kneecap), *Zu San Li* (St 36), and *Jue Gu* (GB 39) mainly treat atony (and) *bi* paralysis of the lower limbs. *Jie Xi* (St 41), *Kun Lun* (Bl 60), *Shang Qiu* (Sp 5), and *Qiu Xu* (GB 40) mainly treat ankle joint pain. *Tai Chong* (Liv 3), *Zu Lin Qi* (GB 41), *Ba Feng* (extra points), and *Qi Duan* (extra point, location unknown) mainly treat swelling, pain, and numbness of the foot and toes.

To promote lactation: *Ru Gen* (St 18), *Shan Zhong* (CV 17), *Shao Ze* (SI 1), and *Zu San Li* (St 36). Mainly treats postpartum insufficient lactation.

To combat consumption (pulmonary tuberculosis): *Zhong Fu* (Lu 1), *Fei Shu* (Bl 13), *Gao Huang Shu* (Bl 43), *Po Hu* (Bl 42), *Bai Lao* (extra point), *Jie Hu Xue* (Tuberculosis Point, extra point), *Zu San Li* (St 36), *Si Hua* (Four Flowers, *i.e.*, Bl 17 and 18), *Huan Men* (extra point, location unknown), and *Da Zhui* (GV 14). Mainly treats pulmonary tuberculosis.

To disperse inflammation: For tonsillitis, pharyngitis, and laryngitis, *Qu Chi* (LI 11), *He Gu* (LI 4), and *Tian Tu* (CV 22). For otitis media, *Er Men* (TH 21), *Ting Gong* (SI 19), *Ting Hui* (GB 2), *Yi Feng* (TH 17), *Zhong Zhu* (TH 3), *Wai Guan* (TH 5), *Yang Ling Quan* (GB 34), and *Qiu Xu* (GB 40). For treating acute appendicitis, *Shang Ju Xu* (St 37), *Zu San Li* (St 36), *Lan Wei Xue* (extra point), *Tian Shu* (St 25), and *Qu Chi* (LI 11). For treating rheumatoid arthritis, *Jian Yu* (LI 15), *Qu Chi* (LI 11), *He Gu* (LI 4), *Huan Tiao* (GB 30), *Yang Ling Quan* (GB 34), *Jue Gu* (GB 39), *Feng Shi* (GB 31), *Zu San Li* (St 36), *Xi Yan* (St 35), and *Shen Shu* (Bl 23).

To terminate malaria: *Da Zhui* (GV 14), *Tao Dao* (GV 10), *Cong Gu* (extra point, located below the spinous process of C6), *Zhi Yang* (GV 9), *Jian Shi* (Per 5), *Hou Xi* (SI 3), *Gan Shu* (Bl 18), *Dan Shu* (Bl 19), *Fu Liu* (Ki 7), *He Gu* (LI 4), and *Zu San Li* (St 36). Mainly treats malarial disease.

To recede jaundice: *Zhi Yang* (GV 9), *Wang Gu* (SI 4), *Yang Gang* (Bl 48), *Dan Shu* (Bl 19), *Ri Yue* (GB 24), *Yang Ling Quan* (GB 34), *Hou Xi* (SI 3), *Yin Ling Quan* (Sp 9), *Pi Shu* (Bl 20), *Lao Gong* (Per 8), *Yong Quan* (Ki 1), *Zhong Wan* (CV 12), and *San Yin Jiao* (Sp 6). Mainly treats jaundice.

To lift the fallen: Needle *Ti Tuo Xue* (Lift Prolapse Point, extra point, located 4 *cun* lateral to CV 4), *Zi Gong Xue* (Fetal Palace Point, extra point, located 3 *cun* lateral to CV 3), and *Hui Yin* (CV 1). Moxa *Qi Hai* (CV 6) and *Bai Hui* (GV 20). Mainly treats uterine prolapse.

6

Composing an Acupuncture Formula

In general, one should try to implement their treatment with as few individual insertions as possible since most patients are naturally acrophobic to some degree. It is my belief that in acupuncture one should strive for the elegance of simplicity while still achieving the proper therapeutic results. In most cases, a well thought out TCM acupuncture treatment should not require more than eight points needled bilaterally. If more than eight points are selected during a single treatment, it is my opinion that:

1) the case is unusually complicated

2) the practitioner has not clarified their diagnosis based on understanding the disease mechanism, or

3) they have not prioritized their treatment goals in terms of a discrimination of *ben* and *biao*, root and branch

This means that they have not clarified for themselves what needs to be treated first and why, what second and why, etc. Therefore, the practitioner should think deeply about the problem at hand and try to pierce the heart of the matter so that, through indirect treatment, one point or one treatment may accomplish several goals simultaneously.

When selecting both the commanding and supplementary points of a formula, the practitioner must take into account not only each point's functions but also their individual characteristics. These characteristics include the channel upon which they are located, their empirically verified symptomatic indications, and any special categories to which they may belong. These categories include the five *shu* or transport points, the *bei shu* or back transport points, the front *mu* or alarm points, the eight *hui* or meeting points of the tissues, the meeting points of the eight extraordinary vessels, the *luo* points, *yuan* source points, *xi* cleft points, entry and exit points, lower *he* sea points, window of the sky points, and crossing points. Point selection based on each of these categories is also discussed in Mark Seem's *Acupuncture Energetics*.[21]

Channel Puncture

Jing ci means to needle points along a channel. This is one of the most important principles of point selection. According to this principle, one selects one or more points along a channel based on either the pathology manifesting along the course of that channel or the pathology being due to an imbalance in the viscus or bowel connected with that channel. In the first case, one might needle *Jian Yu* (LI 15) for shoulder pain along the *yang ming* portion of the shoulder but *Jian Liao* (TH 14) for shoulder pain more on the *shao yang*. In the second case, one might pick a hand *tai yin* point to treat a respiratory problem since the hand *tai yin* pertains to the lungs.

Ju ci means contralateral puncture or needling the opposite side upon which the pathology manifests. This principle is still a variety of *jing ci* in that one discriminates what channel is affected and needles a point or points unilaterally on the same channel on the opposite and ostensibly unaffected side. This is sometimes also referred to as needling the left to treat the right (*yi zuo zhi you*)

---

[21] Seem, Mark, *Acupuncture Energetics, A Workbook for Diagnosis and Treatment*, Thorsons Publishing Group, Rochester, VT, 1987

and needling the right to treat the left (*yi you zhi zuo*). This method is only used when treating one-sided pathologies. It is based on a basic yin/yang reciprocal relationship. If one side is replete, the other must be vacuous. By treating the opposite side, one supplements the vacuity by attracting the qi from the replete side. The net result is then left/right balance. This is a very sophisticated method of point selection which, when it works, often effects a cure with but one needle and one treatment. Often the *luo* points are the points selected for contralateral puncture. Other methods of point selection based on distant puncture (*yuan dao ci*) are puncturing below to treat above (*shang bing xia zhi*), such as choosing *Nei Ting* (St 44) to treat epistaxis, and puncturing above to treat below (*xia bing shang zhi*), such as choosing *Bai Hui* (GV 20) to treat rectal prolapse.

When selecting points along the corresponding (affected) channel (*xun jing qu xue*), one should always remember that the hand and foot channels of a single division (*tai yang, shao yang*, etc.) should be seen as a single channel. That is why *Nei Ting* on the foot *yang ming* can treat a problem of the nose which is traversed by the hand *yang ming*. That is also why it is important for Western acupuncturists to learn this system of naming and referring to the twelve main channels (*shi er zheng jing*) which then become the six channels or *liu jing*.

Symptomatic Indications

As far as symptomatic indications for the various points are concerned, a number of English language texts list these. Of these, *Essentials of Chinese Acupuncture; Acupuncture: A Comprehensive Text;* and *Fundamentals of Chinese Acupuncture* are the three standard sources. However, the first two of these texts describe only the most important indications and also only those indications which can be described in Western medical nomenclature. In my opinion, this is a mistake and I refer the practitioner to the point indications given in Felix Mann's *The Treatment of Disease by Acupuncture.*[22] These specifically Chinese medical indications are based on the *Zhen Jiu Da Cheng (The Great Compendium of Acupuncture/Moxibustion).*[23]

Although Felix Mann has added some obviously modern Western medical indications, such as carbon monoxide poisoning for *Tian Fu* (Lu 3), these additions are easy to identify. I recommend this source of point indications because it is based on a mature acupuncture classic written prior to the advent of modern Western medicine's deleterious impact on Chinese medicine and also because it lists a number of symptoms which, in my experience, patients do experience but which have no technical Western medical name. A feeling of energy rising to the top of the body,[24] a constant desire or need to stretch,[25] feeling as if one eye had been pulled out,[26] or feeling as if energy under high tension shoots up and down[27] are all possible human experiences which modern Western medicine does not describe or treat but Chinese acupuncture does. Likewise, the supplementary point indications in *Fundamentals of Chinese Acupuncture* also seem to be based primarily on the *Zhen Jiu Da Cheng.*

---

[22] Mann, *op.cit.*

[23] Yang Ji-zhou, *Zhen Jiu Da Cheng (The Great Compendium of Acupuncture/Moxibustion)*, 1601

[24] Mann, *op.cit.*, p. 4

[25] *Ibid.*, p.6

[26] *Ibid.*, p. 11

[27] *Ibid.*, p. 11

When choosing acupuncture points based on the lists of points correlated with treatment principles in the preceding chapter, it is extremely important that one not rely totally on these principles alone. One must also assess:

1) if the points affect the channels traversing the affected area

2) if the points are also known empirically to effectively treat the symptoms at hand

Selection of points based on a combination of therapeutic principles, channels, and empirical indications is the basis for rationally composing an acupuncture treatment. All three of these methods of point selection should concur when deciding upon a point or combination of points in TCM acupuncture.

A Shi Points

We should also not forget Sun Si-miao's advice never to forget to needle any *a shi* points when treating pain locally. *A shi* points may or may not be recognized, named and numbered acupuncture points on a channel. They are *de facto* points, however, due to their proximity to the pathology and the fact that they are abnormally sore or painful to palpation. According to the dicta, "If there is free flow there is no pain; if there is pain there is no free flow" and "One hundred diseases arise from (disorders of) the qi," draining *a shi* points often spells the difference between success and failure in the acupuncture treatment of pain.

The named and numbered points are theoretically where the qi and blood can best be adjusted, but *a shi* points are the actual location of blockage and stagnation. For more information on the role of needling *a shi* points in the treatment of chronic pain, the reader is referred to Mark Seem's *A New American Acupuncture: Acupuncture Osteopathy*.[28] This book also exemplifies a rational approach to the selection of acupuncture points based not so much on TCM therapeutic principles but on palpation.

Recapitulation

Having made an individual diagnosis according to the rubric of Chinese medicine and having formulated the heteropathic principles necessary to rebalance the imbalance implied by the TCM pattern discrimination, one selects several main points to rectify the situation in principle while at the same time understanding 1) why each point functions the way it does based on the point's individual characteristics or category, and 2) its indications. These several main points, which typically are distant from the site of the pathology, should be supplemented by one or more local points adjacent to the pathology. One may think of the main points as the transmitter of the message and the local points as the receiver.

The combination of distant main, energetic points and local, supplementary and symptomatic points is the key to the creation of a successful acupuncture formula according to Traditional Chinese Medicine or TCM.

The more painful and acute a situation is, the more local points should be used. This is based on the principle, "Treat the *biao* or branch in acute cases." The more chronic and less painful a disease is, typically the less local and symptomatic points are used. This is based on the principle, "Treat the *ben* or root in chronic cases." However, in modern clinical practice, one typically treats

---

[28] Seem, Mark, *A New American Acupuncture: Acupuncture Osteopathy*, Blue Poppy Press, Boulder, CO, 1993

114

both *ben* and *biao* to some extent at the same time.

As an example of this method of point formulation, let us take a patient who presents with a running nose, sneezing, a slight fever, but no presence of sweat, fear of chill (*wu feng*, *i.e.*, fear of catching a chill), a headache in the back of the neck, stiff, achy shoulders and neck, a thin, white tongue coating, and a floating, somewhat tight pulse. These various signs and symptoms began the night before after being caught out in the wind and rain. The floating, tight pulse, absence of pathological changes in the tongue, recent onset, absence of perspiration, fear of wind, and stiff musculature all point to an external invasion in the exterior. Fear of wind and the fact that the symptoms manifest primarily in the upper body suggest pathologic wind. The tight pulse suggests pathologic cold. The fever without perspiration and the achy musculature show that the *wei qi* has become obstructed and that the pores are closed by the pathogen. Since the lungs are the tender viscus and florid canopy of the other viscera, it is the viscus most susceptible to external invasion. The sneezing shows that the lung qi is counterflowing upward and runny nose shows that the lung qi is not depurating and diffusing the qi and body fluids.

Based on the above diagnosis, the therapeutic principles are to relieve the exterior or to cause diaphoresis, to expel the wind and scatter the cold, and to diffuse, depurate, and downbear the lung qi.

The acupuncture treatment in turn based on these principles is to needle with draining method *He Gu* (LI 4), *Lie Que* (Lu 7), *Feng Men* (Bl 12), *Fei Shu* (Bl 13), *Feng Chi* (GB 20), and *Ying Xiang* (LI 20). *Lie Que* expels wind, relieves the exterior, and diffuses and downbears the lung qi. When combined with *He Gu*, these two points relieve the exterior, cause diaphoresis, and remove obstruction to the lung qi. *He Gu* alone additionally scatters cold and removes obstruction to the defensive qi in the tendinomuscular and skin layer. *Fei Shu* and *Feng Men* dispel external evils from the exterior and rectify the lung qi. *Feng Chi* dispels wind to relieve headache.

In this case, *Lie Que* is chosen based on channel puncture, since it is the lung viscus which has been affected. *He Gu* and *Ying Xiang* are chosen based on treating the yang (channel) to treat the yin. Also, it is the hand *yang ming* which traverses the nose. *Feng Men* and *Feng Chi* are both wind points. Therefore, one can discern in this treatment a number of inter-relationships between these six points, most of which are described under the functions of several of the two point combinations listed above. The diagram below hints at some of these relationships.

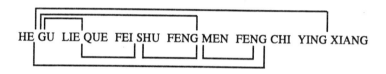

First, the points comprising this formula embody the requisite therapeutic principles for rebalancing the disharmony stated in the name of the pattern discrimination. Secondly, these points comprehensively treat each and every one of the patient's symptoms. And third, each point chosen has a relationship in principle with one or more of the other points. Thus, there is a cohesion to this treatment. Such cohesion and synergism is the hallmark of a formula as opposed to merely a collection of points. There is artistry to the composition of a TCM formula.

After creating such a formula, the beginner should also go back and explain to themselves, as we have done above, why each point has been chosen. This is called *point rationalization*. Each point should have been picked according to rationally arrived at

116

principles through the logical manipulation of the theories and technical terms of TCM. Although this process may seem unnecessarily labored, it is, in my opinion, the quickest way to develop real accuracy and proficiency in writing TCM acupuncture prescriptions.

Usually, more than one acupuncture treatment is necessary to effect a cure in the majority of cases. Each successive time the patient returns, the practitioner should check again the patient's current signs and symptoms, pulse and tongue. As these change and as the TCM pattern diagnosis likewise changes, the treatment should also change. In some cases, it may only be the supplementary points which change. In other cases, because of the evolution of the pattern diagnosis, an entirely different set of main points may have to be formulated. If the symptoms are alleviated but the root remains, one may delete the local points of symptomatic action, retaining the main points of metabolic action.

7

Acupuncture Administration

O nce one has selected the points necessary to redress the imbalance implied in the patient's TCM pattern diagnosis, the practitioner must next implement the manipulation of the qi at these points. According to Wang Le-ting,

> Once a disease has set in, it can be none other than replete, vacuous, or a combination of the two. According to the principle, "If vacuous, supplement; if replete, drain", for vacuity patterns we should supplement and for repletion, drain. For combinations of the two, the vacuities should be supplemented, while the repletions should be drained. Logically, there is no such thing as neither repletion nor vacuity, for, in that case, yin and yang would be balanced, the patient would be normal, and there would be no need for acupuncture.[29]

This means that the practitioner should have a clear and exact idea of what each point is meant to do. It is meant to either supplement vacuity or drain repletion. This clarity of intention is the first and foremost step in achieving supplementation and draining with acupuncture. As with the above steps in the methodology we are presenting, the practitioner should note on the patient's chart which of these two general goals is meant to be achieved at each

---

[29] Wang Le-ting, *Jin Zhen Wang Le Ting*, (*Golden Needle Wang Le-ting*), Beijing, 1984, trans. by Michael Helme, excerpted in "Wang Le-ting on Acupuncture" by Bob Flaws, *Timing and the Times, op.cit.*, p.138

point. *Zhen ci bu xie* means supplementation and draining through the insertion of needles.

Shou Fa or Hand Technique

Exactly how one supplements or drains with needles is a subject of much controversy. One can find various, diametrically opposed techniques claiming to achieve the same effect. In my opinion, whatever technique is chosen should be supported by the logic of TCM theory *and* the practitioner should have great faith in that technique. For instance, Wang Le-ting used a supplementation and draining technique based on the clockwise and counterclockwise rotation of the needle. As his professional biographer notes:

> Dr. Wang works strictly according to where the fourteen channels arise and their direction of flow as well as the upbearing yin/downbearing yang rationale to carry out supplementation and drainage. When the selection of light, medium, or heavy manipulation is added, it completes an easy to perform method that achieves good results in supplementing vacuity and draining repletion. He rarely uses or supports other fancy hand techniques or tries to explore other systems. Rather, he consistently discriminates according to vacuity and repletion and clearly separates whether to supplement or drain as well as how much stimulation to use.[30]

In other words, Wang Le-ting, in surveying the various available techniques for supplementing and draining with acupuncture, selected a method he felt was supported by sound theoretical principles. Then he employed this method with great faith, not looking here, there, or everywhere. He then achieved good clinical results which empirically confirmed the validity of his technique, thus instilling even greater faith. Dr. Wang employed this technique on every point needled after having clarified what

---

[30] *Ibid.*, p. 139

needed to be supplemented and what drained. Up until his death a few of years ago, Dr. Wang was one of the greatest contemporary acupuncturists in northern China.

Classical Methods of Supplementation and Drainage

I suggest the following classical supplementation and draining techniques. The first is called supplementation and draining by opening and closing (*kai he bu xie*). In order to supplement vacuity, one covers the hole upon withdrawing the needle. This insures that no righteous qi escapes from the point upon withdrawal. The door is closed behind the needle, shutting the righteous qi within. To drain evil qi, one leaves the hole from which the needle has been withdrawn open or uncovered. One can even enlarge the hole by rotating the needle in a wide arc upon withdrawal. This opens the door from which evil qi may depart from the body.

The second method is called supplementation and draining by lifting and thrusting (*ti cha bu xie*). If one emphasizes repeatedly pushing the needle down into the point, this is supplementation. If one emphasizes repeatedly pulling the needle up, from deep to shallow, this is drainage. In the first case, one is pushing the *wei* or yang qi down into the *ying* in order to catalyze its growth. This is based on the principle that yang quickens and transforms the yin. In the second, one is again trying to pump or pull out from deep to superficial and ultimately out of the body some evil or pathogenic qi.

The third method is called supplementation and draining by twirling and twisting (*nian zhuan bu xie*). This can be interpreted in two different ways. On the one hand, it can refer to twisting the needle in a yin or yang direction a certain yin or yang number of

121

times, such as Dr. Wang Le-ting and Miriam Lee[31] advocate. However, the specifics of this method are widely varied and disputed. The other interpretation of this phrase is that strong stimulation, for instance through twirling, is draining, while light stimulation is supplementing. This is based on the idea that light stimulation attracts the righteous qi to the point. Whereas, strong stimulation disperses the evil qi like spurring a horse.

The fourth method is called supplementation and draining by meeting and following (*ying sui bu xie*). This means that if the needle is slanted against the flow of the channel according to the chest to hand, hand to head, head to foot, and foot to chest flow of qi, this is draining. If the needle is slanted in the flow of the channel, this is called following and is supplementing.

The fifth method is called supplementation and draining by exhaling and inhaling (*hu xi bu xie*). In order to supplement, one inserts the needle when the patient is exhaling and withdraws the needle when the patient is inhaling. This is based on the fact that, as one exhales, the qi of the entire body expands and moves therefore from deep to superficial. The practitioner then contacts this qi in the yang or superficial region and leads it down into the yin or interior. As one inhales, the qi of the body contracts. If one withdraws the needle during the inhalation, the righteous qi tends to stay deep and will not follow the needle to the surface. Drainage is just the opposite. By inserting during an inhalation, the needle plunges deep into the *ying*. By withdrawing during an exhalation, one blows the evil qi to the exterior following along the track of the needle. Most modern sources explain this process

---

[31] Lee, Miriam, *Insights of a Senior Acupuncturist*, Blue Poppy Press, Boulder, CO, 1992

just the opposite.[32] However, I feel that once one understands the bodily rise and fall of the qi coordinated with exhalation and inhalation, the classical approach is logical.

> (In order to drain,) push the needle in and turn it at the beginning of the inspiration and pull it out slowly at the beginning of the expiration. In order to supplement, it is simply necessary to reach the exterior qi in the skin. Push the needle in at the beginning of the expiration and pull it out at the beginning of the inspiration...[33]

Those with *qi gong* or *gong fu* experience will be able to understand this easily.

The sixth method is called supplementation and draining by swift and mild (insertion) (*ji xu bu xie*). This means that one supplements by inserting the needle slowly and withdrawing it swiftly. Once again, one is attempting to lead the yang qi from the exterior to the interior so that yang can quicken and transform the yin and then leave that qi deep. In order to drain, one inserts the needle deeply quite swiftly. This is again like spurring a horse or throwing a firecracker into the midst of a crowd. Then one leads out the evil qi by slowly withdrawing the needle, leading the evil qi to and out the exterior.

All these methods are essentially based on the concept of three (stratum) puncture (*san ci*). According to this theory, the depth of each point is divided into heaven (shallow), human (medium), and earth (deep) layers. The heavenly layer corresponds to the flow of the *wei yang*, the earthly layer corresponds to the flow of the *ying*

---

[32] For instance, *Chinese-English Terminology of Traditional Chinese Medicine*, *op.cit.*, p. 464

[33] *Huang Di Nei Jing, Su Wen, (Yellow Emperor's Internal Classic, Simple Questions)*, Chapter 27

xue. All the above methods are designed to either 1) lead yang qi deep to quicken and transform the yin in order to supplement or 2) to scatter and lead out the evil qi from deep to superficial in order to disperse.

There are two further needle techniques which are based on the above three (stratum) puncture principle. These are meant to warm and to cool respectively. The first is called *shao shan huo* (setting the mountain on fire).[34] It is for calorification or warming. The practitioner inserts the needle superficially into the heavenly layer. He or she twists the needle nine times and then proceeds down to the human layer. Again the needle is twisted nine times. Finally, one proceeds to the earthly or deep layer and again twists the needle nine times. The needle is then quickly withdrawn to the heavenly layer and the entire process is repeated three times.

The second method for cooling or refrigerating is called cooling like a clear night sky (*tou tian liang*). Here, the needle is thrust quickly and deeply into the earthly layer. The needle is twisted six times and slowly withdrawn up to the human layer. Again it is twisted six times and slowly withdrawn to the heavenly layer. It is twisted six times and then it is thrust quickly down into the earthly layer again. This process is also repeated a total of three times.

In actuality, these two methods are simply species of supplementation and draining. In the first, one is again leading yang qi deep to quicken and transform the *yin ying*. In the second, one is attempting to pull out the evil hot qi to and then from the exterior. However, experiments in China have verified that these

---

[34] In the fall, Chinese farmers burn the straw in the fields. This is called setting the mountain on fire.

methods are capable of changing the temperature within the points and channels.[35]

In clinical practice, one can use all or most of these methods at the same time. They are in no way mutually exclusive. One should select several of them depending upon the TCM pattern diagnosis and the nature and anatomy of the point. For instance, in order to supplement, one can use gentle and slow insertion, three (stratum) puncture, mild manipulation, speedy withdrawal, and can cover the hole all during the same treatment. In addition, if one intends to retain the needle passively, one can also slant the needle in the flow of the channel.

To drain, one can combine just the opposite techniques. At shallow points, such as *Lie Que* (Lu 7), slanting the needle to meet or follow may be the primary method of supplementing or draining. One can also bleed to evacuate to and from the exterior a repletion or one can use moxibustion to scatter cold, warm the channels, and supplement vacuity. Using appropriate *shou fa* or hand technique, one can also drain a point and then immediately supplement it if a point calls for both drainage and supplementation. For instance, according to Miriam Lee, the lungs typically need to be cleared of retained evil heat. This heat is often vacuity heat. Therefore, before the lungs can or should be supplemented, this heat needs to be cleared. If one does not drain evils before attempting to supplement the righteous, one may inadvertently boost the evils.[36]

---

[35] See the *American Journal of Acupuncture*, published in Capitola, CA, for abstracts of Chinese articles concerning the laboratory testing of acupoints and needling techniques.

[36] Lee, *op.cit.*, p. 54-55

De Qi

However, before any manipulation of the qi at a point can be accomplished, one must first *de qi* or obtain the qi. According to TCM acupuncture, without *de qi*, the needle is not manipulating anything.

> But when one needles, if one does not succeed in attracting the qi to the needle, it is necessary to continue needling without being concerned about the number of times. It is necessary to needle until the qi arrives. The purpose, in fact, of needling is to attract the qi. The sign of its arrival is as visible as the wind which makes the clouds disperse. The sick person will be relieved (if and when the qi arrives.)[37]

The subjective sensations that Chinese practitioners traditionally use to describe the arrival or obtainment of qi are distention, heaviness, a nervy, electric feeling propagated along the course of the channel, or a sore, crampy feeling. In China, after inserting the needle, one asks, "*You, mai you* (do you have anything or not)?" If the patient says, "*Mai you* (I don't have anything)," the practitioner attempts to *dao qi* or abduct the qi by any of several manipulations. The needle may have been inserted too deep or too shallow or to the right or left of the point. In this case, one must search for the qi. Or the qi may be sluggish and one must simply manipulate the needle more strongly or for a longer duration to coax it to the point. In that case, one must wait for the qi.

Objectively, the practitioner should feel a relatively sudden increase of resistance in the needle when the qi arrives. This is described classically as being similar to a fish taking the hook.

---

[37] *Huang Di Nei Jing, Ling Shu (Yellow Emperor's Internal Questions, Spiritual Pivot)*, Chapter 1

After asking, "*You, mai you,*" the practitioner often also asks, "*Tong, bu tong* (does it hurt or not)?" *Tong* means pain, particularly a sharp, cutting, biting pain. *Tong* suggests that the needle is erroneously positioned and should be repositioned until there is correct *de qi* without *tong* or pain. The type of pain Chinese understand when they use the word *tong* is not a sign of correct *de qi*. Acupuncture should be *bu tong* or painless. However, many Westerners will experience even proper *de qi* as pain. In English, soreness, cramping, and heaviness are species of pain. Whereas, in Chinese, soreness (*suan*) or distention (*zhang*) are *bu tong*.

Palpating to Locate the Points
And the Method of Insertion & Withdrawal

Wang Le-ting recommends the following step by step protocol for locating points and inserting and withdrawing the needles:

Rubbing is the first step in locating a point. According to the position of the point, one should press and rub in the direction of the channel flow. Especially in points on the four limbs, one should be sure to palpate all the muscles and joints in the area. This relaxes and opens the channels while simultaneously allowing the patient to prepare mentally. At the same time, it allows the doctor to make a close inspection of the local area and the patient's body in general.

"Fingering" the point itself is commonly called "pinching the point". (This is the second step in Wang Le-ting's protocol.) After rubbing the general area, the next step is to locate the specific point on the channel. Dr. Wang's method of point location is according to the traditional relationships of the bones and surface anatomy landmarks in a particular area of the body. This is the way most texts commonly describe point locations. However, in a few cases, he has his own location method, such as for *Huan Tiao* (GB 30), *San Jian* (Three Shoulder points, *i.e.*, *Jian Yu* [LI 15], *Jian Liao* [TH 14], and *Jian Nei Ling* [extra point]), *Du Bi* (St 35), etc. After finding

127

the point, he uses the thumbnail of the left hand to draw a cross on the point such that the point of intersection of the two lines lies directly over the heart of the point. Finally, he presses with his finger. Usually the patient will confirm that it is sore or distended.

On the one hand, this fingering method marks the site of insertion. On the other, palpation of the skin and muscle in the area numbs the site a bit and reduces pain on insertion. It also scatters the local qi and blood, thus avoiding damage to the *ying* and *wei*. After locating the point thus, one should next carry out standard antiseptic procedures.

Inserting the needle is the third step. After decades of clinical experience in inserting needles, Dr. Wang consistently uses both hands and is opposed to one-handed insertion. He emphasizes the importance of guiding with the left hand. He feels that with the two-handed insertion the strength is appropriate, the needle is steady, the point is needled precisely, and there is no way to swing to the right or left nor movement up or down to cause the needle to miss its mark. Usually the patient feels no pain this way. As it says in the *Biao You Fu*, "The left hand is heavy and pressing down. This tends to lead the qi towards dispersing. The right hand is light and moves quickly. This is the reason for no pain."

All the time, while inserting, applying hand technique and moving the needle, (Dr. Wang) always strictly follows the rules of protocol according to *Su Wen (Simple Questions), "Zhen Jie Pian (Needling Explained)"*: "The hand is as if grasping a tiger and admiring its strength. The mind cares not for who or what is around. With a settled will observing the patient, one looks neither to the right nor to the left."[38]

As for removing the needle, (Dr. Wang) also does not let this go unnoticed. As it is said in *Su Wen, "Zhen Jie Pian"*, "When evil qi is victorious, then empty it. Remove the needle and do not cover

---

[38] Wang Le-ting, *op.cit.*, p. 137-138

it." When the pathogen is flourishing and the patient is exhibiting repletion symptoms, do not cover the hole. Rather, let the pathogen drain out. If the righteous is vacuous, then slowly remove the needle and quickly cover the hole, thus allowing the righteous qi to fill in and avoiding any further damage from the outside. When removing the needle, first spin it a little in both directions to loosen the surrounding tissue. This avoids a stuck needle and prevents damage to the environs. Afterwards, proceed according to the above instructions for either supplementing or draining. One should try to start properly and finish properly making the treatment reach and maintain a plateau through a set period of time. To cultivate discipline, one should oppose the practice of withdrawing needles as if pulling onions.[39]

Propagation of Sensation

According to Chinese TCM acupuncture practitioners, it is particularly important in the treatment of pain that one obtains definite *de qi* and that the qi sensation is propagated to the affected area. If one does not get any radiation of sensation, then either the qi has not been obtained or else the qi is not being mobilized in the proper direction. In some cases, there may be *de qi* but the qi sensation is radiating in the opposite direction along the channel from the sight of the pain. In that case, if the practitioner applies finger pressure directly behind the point of insertion and then manipulates the needle, the qi will propagate along the channel in the desired direction. For instance, if, when needling *Wai Guan* (TH 5) for pain on the *shao yang* portion of the shoulder, the qi sensation extends into the wrist but not proximally, by pressing distal to the insertion while at the same time manipulating the needle, one can make the qi ascend and extend the sensation to the site of the problem.

---

[39] *Ibid.*, p. 139

Needle Retention

It has become routine practice in the West to passively retain needles for 20 minutes. However, as a routine, this has led to, in my opinion, sloppy acupuncture. I agree with Dr. Max Wu of San Francisco that such routine retention commonly is used in place of definite *de qi* and the clear performance of *bu fa* (supplementing technique) and *xie fa* (draining technique). As Drs. Wu, Miriam Lee, Cheng Tan-an, and So Tin-yau[40] all emphasize, one must first obtain the qi. Then one should manipulate the needle to affect either *bu fa* or *xie fa*. Having done what one intended, one can remove the needles immediately unless one chooses to retain them *for a specific purpose*. In other words, there is nothing sacrosanct about 20 minutes passive retention. It does not necessarily take 20 minutes to get a good *bu* or *xie* effect.

If a treatment has been well crafted and administered, *i.e.*, the right points have been needled the right way with the right amount of stimulation, the patient should experience deep relaxation, both muscular and mental, a deepening of respiration, possibly a healthy hunger, and a profoundly relaxed but alert energy when the treatment is over. This is so whether the treatment was meant to achieve supplementation or drainage. This is because a good treatment re-establishes balance and these are the signs of the body's being at ease. If one chooses too many points, needles too forcefully, or leaves the needles in place for too long, this may drain the righteous qi, thus leaving the patient exhausted after the treatment. Such exhaustion is typically the sign of a poorly thought-out and executed treatment.

---

[40] So Tin-yau (James), *Treatment of Disease with Acupuncture*, Vol. II, Paradigm Publications, Brookline, MA, 1987, p. 19

Here in the West, however, routinely retaining the needles for 20 minutes does have one good effect. Since we live in a very stressful society and environment, lying down for 20 minutes in the middle of the day is usually beneficial for the majority of Westerners. But, when time does not permit, one should be able to do what needs to be done in far less time. One should not think that all that needs to be done is to put the needles in and leave them for 20 minutes as if one were putting a pie in the oven.

Typically in Chinese acupuncture clinics, if one chooses to needle both ventral and dorsal points, the ventral points are needled first and retained. Then the dorsal points are inserted one by one, *de qi* is obtained, *shou fa* is administered, and the needle is immediately removed. This is to save time since a 20 minute retention on both sides tends to be inconvenient for both the patient and practitioner and is, in fact, unnecessary.

Number of Treatments

Whether one finds the qi shallow or deep, whether the qi moves quickly or slowly, and how many points and how many treatments are necessary all depend upon a number of variables. In general, if a patient gets good *de qi* and especially radiation to the affected area, a better result will be obtained. Some patients are more sensitive and receptive to acupuncture than others. For instance, thin people tend to be more sensitive to acupuncture than heavy-set or obese people, although also more skittish and needle shy. This is because their relative proportion of qi to substance or yang to yin is high. During warm days and warm seasons, the qi in everyone tends to be shallower and quicker. In China, more patients seek acupuncture treatment in the spring and summer than in fall and winter.

131

When it is warm and fine weather, the blood in humans moves rapidly (and) the qi is superficial. When the weather is cold and gloomy, the blood moves less rapidly (and) the qi is deep.[41]

Therefore, the number of treatments necessary to affect a cure in any given patient is a function of several things: 1) the sensitivity and receptivity of the patient to acupuncture, 2) the time of year and weather during acupuncture treatment, 3) the correctness of the diagnosis and, therefore, the appropriateness of the points selected and the methods of their manipulation, 4) the length of time that the patient has suffered from the disease, 5) the severity of the disease, 6) the rapport between the patient and practitioner, and 7) the strength of the practitioner's qi. All these factors play a part in any given patient's response to acupuncture treatment. However, in general, the longer or more serious a disease is, the more treatments are typically necessary to affect a cure. Acute conditions or relatively simple conditions may only require 1-3 treatments. But chronic conditions may require 10's of treatments over many weeks or months. And progressive degenerative conditions may require regular acupuncture over a period of years to either maintain the patient in remission or at least keep the disease from progressing further.

Frequency of Treatment

In China, where treatment is largely paid for by the government and where time off to go to the clinic is freely given and also paid for, acupuncture is most often administered 3 times per week or every other day with 2 days off over the weekend. After 10-15 sessions in such close proximity, constituting one course of treatment, patients are advised to wait 1 week before commencing a second such course of treatment. As mentioned above, for

---

[41] *Huang Di Nei Jing, Su Wen*, Chapter 25

chronic problems, often 10-20 treatments are necessary to markedly ameliorate a problem. Whereas, acute diseases may often be cured with but 1-2 treatments. For acute emergency conditions, as many as 3 treatments may be given per day.

Here in the America where economic necessities require each treatment to cost literally scores of times more than in China and where neither our government, our insurance, nor our employers will typically pick up the bill, many practitioners feel their patients cannot afford so many treatments in such close proximity. Therefore, the once weekly treatment has become the norm in many clinics.

However, it is my experience that in acute situations, during certain periods of time in cyclic conditions, and at the beginning of a course of treatment, more closely spaced treatments often spell the difference between success and failure with acupuncture. For instance, in the treatment of premenstrual breast distention and pain which worsens before each period, 3 treatments given every other day during the week of the premenstruum are more effective than once weekly treatments throughout the cycle. Or, in the case of acute morning sickness, daily or twice daily treatments may be necessary for the first 3-5 days of treatment and if treatment is given that often, truly remarkable results may be obtained. For the practitioner, the single most important issue must be the alleviation of the patient's pain. This means that treatment should be given as frequently as necessary regardless of cost.

Prohibitions to Needling

The prohibitions to puncturing *(jin ci)* include various forbidden points and also needling when the patient is drunk, famished, exhausted, over-stuffed, upset, or after sex. These last six are all situations when the patient's yin and yang are more than normally out of balance. During these times, one might further imbalance the patient in an unforeseen way due to the abnormality of their qi flow. In particular, when a patient is fatigued from hunger, exhaustion, or sex, it is important not to disperse any further righteous qi. Patients who are excessively hungry before a treatment may be given some fruit juice to drink or a piece of fruit to eat. They should then be allowed to wait 15-20 minutes before receiving their acupuncture treatment.

Traditionally in premodern times, acupuncture prohibitions also included treating during the dark of the new moon and at the full moon, during thunder storms, at the equinoxes and solstices, during eclipses, floods, and other natural calamities and anomalies in the weather. These were likewise believed to be times when the macrocosmic yin and yang were in great flux. Because humans exist within heaven and earth, it was believed that the qi in human bodies was also likely to be unpredictably out of balance at such times. Therefore, the acupuncturist was counselled to wait until the macrocosmic qi of heaven and earth had returned to relative normalcy before attempting to balance the qi within their patient. Whether or not such prohibitions are still valid today is a subject open to debate. The reader will have to decide such questions for themself. On the one hand, attention to such prohibitions does reinforce a closer integration of person and their environment. On the other, they may only be cultural beliefs unsupported by clinical evidence.

Older practitioners are often heard to say that, for them, there are no forbidden points. This means that most of the points that are listed in the premodern texts are forbidden to needling only under certain circumstances or when needled in a certain way. These prohibitions are meant primarily for beginners. As one becomes more experienced, these prohibitions merely become reminders to proceed with care. In particular, there are a number of points which are forbidden to needle during pregnancy. This means that they are forbidden to use unless they are specifically indicated for the treatment of some disease condition during pregnancy. For instance, *Zu San Li* (St 36) is forbidden during pregnancy. However, if the woman is suffering from nausea during pregnancy (*ren shen e zu*) due to disharmony of the stomach, then one can needle *Zu San Li* to harmonize the stomach and downbear counterflow. What is forbidden is to needle *Zu San Li* during pregnancy without symptoms of a spleen and stomach disorder or insufficiency of qi.

The management of acupuncture accidents, such as needle shock (*yun zhen*) and bent and broken needles, is covered in other standard texts.[42]

Some Western acupuncturists feel that a wrong or improperly executed acupuncture treatment will have no deleterious effect on the patient, that acupuncture is a fairly benign and minimal intervention, that it can point out to the organism how to correct itself, but, should it be wrong, the organism will disregard this input. Although there is a certain amount of truth in these beliefs about this art, I do not entirely agree with them. My clinical experience suggests that improper acupuncture can make someone sicker or experience more pain. In such cases, either the diagnosis was right but the points were wrong, or the diagnosis and points were right but the *shou fa* or hand technique was wrong. As Zhang Chen-chun wrote in the nineteenth century:

> The abuse of the acupuncture needle amounts to treating human existence as though it were a child's plaything. Anyone who is

---

[42] *Acupuncture: A Comprehensive Text, op.cit.*, p. 414-417

aware of the gravity of the act of healing will know what I am talking about.[43]

---

[43] Zhang Chen-jun, *Li Cheng An Mo Yao Shu*, 1880, trans. by Pierre Huard and Ming Wong, excerpted in *Oriental Methods of Mental and Physical Fitness*, Funk and Wagnals, NY, 1971, p. 146

8

Conclusion

The above step by step methodology of moving from a TCM pattern diagnosis to administering an acupuncture treatment is logically clear cut. At every step, one manipulates the terms of TCM in a conceptually disciplined way to arrive at greater and greater clarity and focus of intention. This step by step methodology is already so clear and apparent in the Chinese language that, in Chinese, one does not need to laboriously spell out this procedure. It is my experience, however, that non-Chinese reading Western practitioners need to learn this conceptual system as a new way of thinking.

In particular, the terms of Chinese medicine are like code ciphers. They are technical terms which have much more specific meanings than most Westerners at first realize. If one manipulates these terms as precisely and as logically as the Chinese, then we can also assume that we will get the same time-tested results. Certainly that is my experience.

I believe that the more we understand and employ Traditional Chinese Medicine as the Chinese do or at least the educated traditional Chinese doctor does, the better will be our clinical results.

About the Author

Bob Flaws, Dipl. Ac., Dipl. C.H., FNAAOM, is an internationally known practitioner, teacher, and writer on acupuncture and Traditional Chinese Medicine. Originally trained in acupuncture by Dr. (Eric) Tao Xi-yu, Bob went on to study acupuncture, *tui na*, and Chinese herbal medicine at the Shanghai College of Traditional Chinese Medicine. Later, Bob was awarded a doctoral degree by Anton Jayasurya of Sri Lanka.

Bob's other credits include founding Blue Poppy Press of which he is the publisher and editor, and helping found the Acupuncture Association of Colorado (AAC) and the Council of Oriental Medical Publishers (COMP). Bob has served on the AAC board of directors for two terms and has been president of the AAC also for two terms. Besides authoring more than 25 books and scores of articles on various topics on Oriental medicine, Dr. Flaws is also author of an NIH-funded protocol for the acupuncture treatment of HIV-related peripheral neuropathy.

English Language Bibliography

Acupuncture Case Histories from China, ed. by Chen Ji-rui & Nissi Wang, Eastland Press, Seattle, 1988

Acupuncture: A Comprehensive Text, Shanghai College of TCM, trans. by John O'Connor & Dan Bensky, Eastland Press, Chicago, 1981

Acumoxatherapy: A Reference & Study Guide, Paul Zmiewski & Richard Feit, Paradigm Publications, Brookline, MA, 1989

Acupuncture: Patterns & Practice, Li Xue-mei & Zhao Jing-yi, Eastland Press, Seattle, 1993

Acupuncture Points: Images & Functions, Arnie Lade, Eastland Press, Seattle, 1989

Chinese Acupuncture and Moxibustion, ed. by Cheng Xin-nong, Foreign Language Press, Beijing, 1987

Chinese-English Terminology of Traditional Chinese Medicine, ed. by Sung J. Liao, Hunan Science and Technology Press, 1983

Dictionary of Traditional Chinese Medicine, ed. by Xie Zhu-fan, The Commercial Press Ltd., Hong Kong, 1984

Essentials of Chinese Acupuncture & Moxibustion, ed. by Cheng Xin-nong, Foreign Language Press, Beijing, 1980

Fundamentals of Chinese Acupuncture, Andrew Ellis, Nigel Wiseman, & Ken Boss, Paradigm Publications, Brookline, MA, 1988

Fundamentals of Chinese Medicine, trans. & ed. by Nigel Wiseman, Andrew Ellis, & Paul Zmiewski, Paradigm Publications, Brookline, MA, 1985

Glossary of Chinese Medical Terms and Acupuncture Points, Nigel Wiseman and Ken Boss, Paradigm Publications, Brookline, MA, 1990

Grasping the Wind: An Exploration of the Meanings of Chinese Acupuncture Point Names, Andrew Ellis, Nigel Wiseman, & Ken Boss, Paradigm Publications, Brookline, MA, 1989

Highlights of Ancient Acupuncture Prescriptions, trans. by Honora Lee Wolfe & Rose Crescenz, Blue Poppy Press, Boulder, CO 1991

How to Write a TCM Herbal Formula, Bob Flaws, Blue Poppy Press, Boulder, CO, 1994

Statements of Fact in TCM, Bob Flaws, Blue Poppy Press, Boulder, CO, 1994

The Essential Book of Traditional Chinese Medicine, Vol. I & II, Liu Yan-chi, trans. by Fang Ting-yu & Chen Lai-di, Columbia University Press, NY, 1988

The Essential of Chinese Diagnostics, Manfred Porkert, Chinese Medicine Publications, Ltd., Zurich, 1983

The Systematic Classic of Acupuncture & Moxibustion: A Translation of Huang-fu Mi's Zhen Jiu Jia Yi Jing, trans. by Yang Shou-zhong & Charles Chace, Blue Poppy Press, Boulder, CO, 1994

Tongue Diagnosis In Chinese Medicine, Giovanni Maciocia, Eastland Press, Seattle, 1987

Web That Has No Weaver, Ted Kaptchuk, Congdon & Weed, NY, 1983

Zang Fu: The Organ Systems of Traditional Chinese Medicine, Jeremy Ross, Churchill Livingstone, Edinburgh, 1988

Index

A

a shi points 113
A New American Acupuncture: Acupuncture Osteopathy 114
abdominal pain 7, 22, 23, 51, 105
abnormal vaginal discharge 7, 41, 65, 91
Acupuncture: A Comprehensive Text 111, 135
Acupuncture Energetics 110
acute lumbar strain 103
amenorrhea 104
angina pectoris 105
ankle, injury of the 103
ankle joint pain 106
aphasia 102
apoplexy 102
appendicitis 96, 105, 106
atony (and) *bi* paralysis of the lower limbs 106
atony pattern 11

B

ba gang 5, 9
ba gang bian zheng 9
Ba Feng (extra points) 106
Ba Xie (extra points) 105
back of the neck pain 105
back transport points 110
Bai Hui (GV 20) 69, 84, 86, 87, 95, 97, 101-103, 107, 111
Bai Lao (extra point) 106
beng lou 23, 101
Bi Guan (St 31) 106
bian zheng lun zhi 8, 9
bing ji 10, 13, 15
bing yin bian zheng 9

bleeding, stop 38, 103
blood division 2, 74, 80
blood, loss of 101
blood pressure, high 104
blood pressure, lower the 104
blood pressure, raise the 104
blood, supplement the 40, 101
boils 104
borborygmus 102
Boss, Ken 1
bowel movements, promote 100
brain, arouse the 38, 102
Brooks, Dennis 3
bu fa 130
buttock pain 105

C

Chang Qiang (GV 1) 89
channel and connecting vessel pattern discrimination 9
channel puncture 110, 116
channels, twelve regular 2
Cheng Fu (Bl 36) 106
Cheng Shan (Bl 57) 89, 102, 103
Cheng Tan-an 130
chest and epigastric distention 102
chest pain 105
Chi Ze (Lu 5) 73, 84, 88, 97, 101, 103
Chinese-English Terminology of Traditional Chinese Medicine 24
Chong Yang (St 42) 50
Chuan Xi (extra point) 101
Ci Liao (Bl 32) 105
clear heat 23, 30-33, 34, 37, 38, 100
cold damage 7
combat consumption 106
conception vessel 70

constructive division 31, 74
contralateral puncture 110, 111
cough and stuffy chest 101
Crescenz, Rose 3
crossing points 110

D

Da Bao (Sp 21) 103
Da Chang Shu (Bl 25) 57, 89, 94, 100
Da Dun (Liv 1) 66, 74, 100
Da Heng (Ki 12) 89, 92
Da Heng (Sp 15) 89, 100
Da Ju (St 27) 90
Da Ling (Per 7) 81, 87, 103, 105
Da Shu (Bl 11) 86, 95, 99
Da Zhong (Ki 4) 60
Da Zhui (GV 14) 69, 82, 94, 100, 105-107
dai xia 7
Dai Mai (GB 26) 65, 91, 95
Dan Shu (Bl 19) 93, 107
de qi 126, 127, 129-131
delivery, delayed 104
delivery, hasten 104
delivery, sluggish 104
dermatology 7
Di Cang (St 4) 48
Di Ji (Sp 8) 52, 104, 105
diarrhea, stop 41, 78, 100
dietary therapy 4
Ding Chuan (extra point) 101
disease diagnosis 6, 8, 18, 19
disease mechanism or dynamic 10
disperse food stagnation 100
disperse inflammation 106
distant puncture 111
downbearing of the turbid 42
draining technique 120, 130
Du Bi (St 35) 103, 127

E

eczema 10
edema, superficial 18
eight principle pattern discrimination 9
eight principles 5, 8, 9
elbow joint pain 105
Ellis, Andrew 1
entry and exit points 110
enuresis 103
epistaxis 73, 103, 111
Er Men (TH 21) 90, 106
Essentials of Chinese Acupuncture 13, 111
exercise 4
external medicine 7

F

Fei Shu (Bl 13) 73, 81, 88, 90, 101, 106, 115
Feng Chi (GB 20) 64, 82, 85, 94, 96, 103, 105, 115
Feng Fu (GV 16) 69, 103
Feng Long (St 40) 50, 78, 85, 93, 97, 100-102, 105
Feng Men (Bl 12) 55, 90, 115
five phase pattern discrimination 9
fluids and humors pattern discrimination 9
food stagnation, disperse 100
forgetfulness 102
four examinations 5, 8, 17, 18
free the vessels 39, 102
fu ke 7, 7
Fu Liu (Ki 7) 60, 74, 81, 88, 92, 96, 99, 107
Fu Tu (St 32) 106
Fundamentals of Chinese Acupuncture 45, 111, 112

furuncles 104

G

Gan Shu (Bl 18) 56, 89, 93, 94, 107
Gao Huang Shu (Bl 43) 58, 106
gastritis 6, 12
Ge Shu (Bl 17) 89, 96, 101-103, 105
Gong Sun (Sp 4) 51, 77, 79, 92, 99, 100, 105
governing vessel 69
Guan Chong (TH 1) 63, 86, 97
Guan Yuan (CV 4) 70, 83, 84, 92, 95, 101, 103
Guan Yuan Shu (Bl 26) 101
Guang Ming (GB 37) 65
Gui Lai (St 29) 49, 87, 94, 104
gynecology 7

H

hand and fingers, numbness of 105
hand technique 120, 125, 128, 135
He Gu (LI 4) 47, 81, 83, 94, 99, 100, 103-107, 115
head pain 105
headache 103, 115, 116
hemiplegia 104
hemorrhoidal bleeding 103
herbal medicine 4
hip joint pain 106
Hou Xi (SI 3) 53, 99, 100, 102, 105, 107
hu xi bu xie 122
Huan Tiao (GB 30) 65, 80, 95, 104, 106, 107, 127
Hui Yin (CV 1) 107

I

immune system 2
infantile paralysis 104
inflammation, disperse 106
internal medicine 7
invigorate yang 40, 101
itching 10

J

jaundice 85, 96, 107
ji xu bu xie 123
Jia Che (St 6) 86, 102, 105
Jia Xi (GB 43) 79
Jian Jing (GB 21) 64, 90, 103
Jian Li (CV 11) 78, 90
Jian Liao (TH 14) 105, 110
Jian Nei Ling (extra point) 105
Jian Shi (Per 5) 61, 78, 82, 86, 94, 100, 102, 107
Jian Yu (LI 15) 48, 83, 104, 105, 107, 110
Jie Hu Xue (Tuberculosis Point, extra point) 106
Jie Xi (St 41) 50, 76, 106
jin ci 133
jin ye bian zheng 9
Jin Jin (extra point) 88
Jin Suo (GV 8) 102
jing ci 110
Jing Gong (Bl 52) 101
Jing Ming (Bl 1) 54, 94, 97
ju ci 110
Ju Gu (LI 16) 105
Ju Que (CV 14) 72, 82, 91, 102
Jue Yin Shu (Bl 14) 102

K

kai he bu xie 121
knee, injury of the 103
Kong Zui (Lu 6) 103
Kuan Gu (Hip Bone, extra point) 103
Kun Lun (Bl 60) 58, 91, 102-106

L

lactation, insufficient 106
lactation, promote 41, 106
Lan Wei Xue (extra point) 105
Lao Gong (Per 8) 62, 82, 87, 99, 107
laryngitis 106
leg pain 105
Li Dui (St 45) 77
Lian Quan (CV 23) 87
Liang Men (St 21) 48, 87, 96
Liang Qiu (St 34) 49
Lie Que (Lu 7) 73, 81, 101, 105, 115, 125
lift the fallen 107
limbs, atony (and) *bi* paralysis of the lower 106
limbs, paralysis of the lower 105, 106
limbs, spasms of the four 102
Ling Tai (GV 10) 91, 103
liu fen bian zheng 9
liu yin 2
lower abdominal pain 7, 22, 23
lumbar and back pain 105
luo points 110, 111
Luo Zhen (extra point) 105

M

malaria 40, 100, 107
malaria, terminate 40, 107
mammary abscess 103
mania and withdrawal 102
Mann, Felix 112
massage therapy 4
meeting points of the eight extraordinary vessels 110
menorrhagia 14
menstrual bleeding, excessive 14, 15
menstrual cycle, shortened 14
menstruation ahead of schedule 8
menstruation, early 22
menstruation, open 104
menstruation, painful 8, 105
Ming Men (GV 4) 69, 83, 101, 105
mouth, dry 22, 104
MS 13
muscular spasticity 15

N

Nao Shu (SI 10) 105
neck pain, back of the 105
neck, wry 105
needle shock 135
nei ke 7
Nei Guan (Per 6) 61, 76, 92, 99, 101, 102, 104, 105
Nei Jing Su Wen 21
Nei Ting (St 44) 51, 81, 84, 85, 94, 100, 105, 111
nephritis 18, 19
neurodermatitis 10
nian zhuan bu xie 121
nue 40, 100
number of treatments 131, 132

O

open menstruation 104
open the portals and utter sound
  102
osteoarthritis 104
otitis media 106
Ou-yang Yi 11

P

palpitations 42, 61, 87, 102
Pang Guang Shu (Bl 28) 57, 88,
  103
pattern diagnosis 5, 15, 17-19, 21,
  42, 117, 119, 125, 137
pattern discrimination 5, 8, 9, 12,
  14-16, 18, 19, 23, 114, 116
pattern discrimination, channel and
  connecting vessel 9
pattern discrimination, disease cause
  9
pattern discrimination, eight principle 9
pattern discrimination, five phase 9
pattern discrimination, fluids and
  humors 9
pattern discrimination, qi and blood
  9
pattern discrimination, six division 9
pattern discrimination, three burners
  9
pattern discrimination, viscera and
  bowels 9
pharyngitis 106
phlegm rheum 6, 11, 12
pi fu ke 7
Pi Shu (Bl 20) 56, 76, 79, 80, 85,
  89, 91, 93, 96, 97, 100-102, 107
PID 7
placenta, retained 64, 104

Po Hu (Bl 42) 106
point rationalization 116
produce saliva and quench thirst
  104
propagation of sensation 129
psoriasis 10
pulmonary tuberculosis 106
purulence 10

Q

qi and blood pattern discrimination
  9
qi dynamic 12, 51
qi shan 7
qi, supplement the 38, 40, 101
qi xue bian zheng 9
Qi Hai (CV 6) 71, 78, 89, 92, 95,
  101, 102, 107
Qi Men (Liv 14) 74, 105
Qin Bo-wei 16
Qiu Xu (GB 40) 93, 103, 105,
  106
Qu Chi (LI 11) 48, 77, 80-83, 93,
  96, 100, 102-107
Qu Quan (Liv 8) 67
Que Pen (St 12) 105
quiet the spirit 40, 42, 82, 102

R

Ran Gu (Ki 2) 74, 92, 104
rectal prolapse 111
rectify the qi 28, 34, 36, 102
redness and inflammation 10
Ren Zhong (GV 26) 70, 77, 85, 96,
  97, 102
resolve toxins 30, 31, 103
rheumatoid arthritis 107
Ri Yue (GB 25) 74
rib pain, upper 105

ribs, injury of the 103
Ru Gen (St 18) 90, 106

S

sacroiliac joint pain 105
san ci 123
san jiao bian zheng 9
San Jiao Shu (Bl 22) 103
San Yin Jiao (Sp 6) 52, 73, 75, 77, 79, 83, 91, 101-105, 107
scaling 10
sciatica 106
setting the mountain on fire 124
seven *shan* 7
Shan Zhong (CV 17) 72, 75, 77, 87, 99, 101, 102, 105, 106
shang han 7
Shang Ju Xu (St 37) 75, 94, 96, 106
Shang Wan (CV 13) 72, 76
Shang Xing (GV 23) 103
Shang Yang (LI 1) 86
shao fu tong 7
shao shan huo 124
Shao Hai (Ht 3) 100, 104, 105
Shao Shang (Lu 11) 47, 84, 86, 97, 100, 105
Shao Ze (SI 1) 53, 84, 87, 106
shen jing xing pi yan 10
Shen Mai (Bl 62) 58, 91
Shen Men (Ht 7) 82, 86, 91, 92, 102, 105
Shen Que (CV 8) 89, 95
Shen Shu (Bl 23) 56, 83, 84, 92, 96, 101, 103, 105, 107
Shen Zhu (GV 12) 91, 94
shi er zheng jing 2, 111
shi zheng 10
Shi Xuan (extra points) 102
shou fa 120, 125, 131, 135

Shou San Li (LI 10) 105
shoulder and arm, injury of the 103
shoulder joint pain 106
Shu Fu (Ki 27) 60
shui zhong 18
Shui Dao (St 28) 49, 104
Shui Fen (CV 9) 71, 79, 90
Shui Quan (Ki 5) 87
si zhen 5
Si Shen Cong (Four Immortals, extra points) 102
sleep, loss of 102
So Tin-yau 130
spasms of the four limbs 102
spasms, relieve 102
Steinway, Nina 3
stomach pain 105
stop pain 105
stranguries, five 7
stroke 97, 101, 104
Su Wen (Simple Questions), "Zhen Jie Pian (Needling Explained)" 128
supplement the blood 40, 101
supplement the qi 38, 40, 101
supplementary points 109, 117
supplementation and draining by swift and mild (insertion) 123
supplementing technique 130
suppuration 10
sweating, start 99
symptomatic indications 110, 111

T

Tai Chong (Liv 3) 67, 74, 76, 79, 90, 93, 94, 102-106
Tai Xi (Ki 3) 59, 73, 83, 84, 92, 96, 102, 104
Tai Yang (extra point) 105
Tai Yuan (Lu 9) 47, 73, 76, 81, 88, 101

tan yin 6, 12
Tao Dao (GV 13) 100
Tao Xi-yu 3
The Great Compendium of Acupuncture/Moxibustion 112
therapeutic principles 4, 21, 23, 24, 42, 45, 114-116
thirst 22, 88, 104
thirst, produce saliva and quench 104
three (stratum) puncture 123-125
three burners pattern discrimination 9
throat, dry 104
throat pain 105
ti cha bu xie 121
Tian Chi (Per 1) 61
Tian Fu (Lu 3) 112
Tian Jing (TH 10) 63, 100, 105
Tian Shu (St 25) 49, 76, 78, 87, 94-96, 100, 100, 104, 105, 107
Tian Tu (CV 22) 73, 75, 85, 87, 94, 102, 105, 106
Tian Zhu (Bl 10) 54, 90, 105
Ting Gong (SI 19) 106
Ting Hui (GB 2) 90, 106
tong jing 8, 41
Tong Li (Ht 5) 53, 102
tonsillitis 106
tooth pain 105
tou tian liang 124
tranquilize one's composure 102
transport points 110

U

upbearing of the pure 42
urinary incontinence 14, 103
urination, disinhibit 103
uterine bleeding 22, 41, 101
uterine prolapse 107

V

viscera and bowels pattern discrimination 9
vomiting 27, 50, 62, 67, 75, 77, 78, 93, 94, 99, 105
vomiting, initiate 99
vomiting, stop 75, 78, 99

W

Wai Guan (TH 5) 63, 82, 94, 100, 106, 129
Wang Gu (SI 4) 107
Wang Le-ting 119-122, 127, 128
warm disease 7, 21, 30, 31
warm the middle and stem yang 101
water swelling 18
wei qi 2, 9, 28, 115
wei qi ying xue bian zheng 9
wei zheng 11-14, 80
Wei Shu (Bl 21) 56, 89, 96
Wei Zhong (Bl 40) 57, 96, 103, 105
wen bing 7
wheezing, stabilize 101
wind, dispel 35, 36, 96, 103, 104
window of the sky points 110
Wolfe, Honora Lee 3
wrist joint, injury of the 103
wry neck 105
wu lin 7
Wu, Max 130
wu xing bian zheng 9
Wu Shu (GB 27) 91

X

xi cleft points 110
Xi Men (Per 4) 61, 87, 105
Xi Yan (St 35) 106, 107

Xi Yang-jiang 3, 45
Xia Guan (St 7) 86, 105
Xia Ju Xu (St 39) 89, 94, 95, 104
Xian Gu (St 43) 82, 84, 100
Xiao Chang Shu (Bl 27) 57, 88, 89, 95
Xiao Shao-qing 99
xie fa 130
Xin Shu (Bl 15) 82, 102, 105
Xing Jian (Liv 2) 67, 74, 78, 79, 85, 92, 93
Xuan Ji (CV 21) 100
Xuan Zhong (aka *Jue Gu*, GB 39) 66, 80, 86, 95
xue fen 2
Xue Hai (Sp 10) 74, 80, 92, 96

Y

Ya Men (GV 15) 102
Yang Gang (Bl 48) 107
Yang Gu (TH 4) 105
Yang Ling Quan (GB 34) 65, 79, 93, 95, 100, 102-107
Yi Feng (TH 17) 64, 86, 90, 106
Yin Bai (Sp 1) 51, 103
Yin Ling Quan (Sp 9) 52, 95, 103, 104, 107
Yin Tang (extra point) 85, 91, 97, 105
ying fen 31
ying sui bu xie 122
ying xie bing 10
Ying Xiang (LI 20) 48, 81, 91, 96, 115
Yong Quan (Ki 1) 59, 85, 102, 104, 107
Yu Ye (extra point) 88
yuan dao ci 111
yuan source points 110
yue jing guo duo 22

yue jing xian qi 8, 22
yun zhen 135

Z

Zan Zhu (Bl 2) 54, 97
Zhang Chen-chun 135
Zhang Men (Liv 13) 78, 85, 101
Zhao Hai (Ki 6) 73, 92, 100, 104, 105
Zhen Jiu Da Cheng 112
zheng 2, 5, 6, 8-15, 18, 24, 25, 80, 111
Zhi Bian (Bl 54) 105, 106
Zhi Gou (TH 6) 63, 75, 80, 83, 94, 100, 105
Zhi Yang (GV 9) 107
Zhi Yin (Bl 67) 104
Zhong Feng (Liv 4) 86
Zhong Fu (Lu 1) 106
Zhong Guo Zhen Jiu Chu Fang Xue 7, 99
Zhong Ji (CV 3) 70, 74, 85, 88, 95, 103
Zhong Wan (CV 12) 71, 75, 77-79, 91-93, 95-97, 99, 101, 105, 107
Zhong Zhu (TH 3) 106
Zhou Jian (tip of the olecranon process) 100
Zu Lin Qi (GB 41) 66, 85, 93, 97, 106
Zu San Li (St 36) 50, 75, 76, 91-93, 95, 99-107, 134

OTHER BOOKS ON CHINESE MEDICINE AVAILABLE FROM BLUE POPPY PRESS

1775 Linden Ave ○ Boulder, CO 80304
For ordering 1-800-487-9296
PH. 303\447-8372 FAX 303\447-0740

THE HEART & ESSENCE Of Dan-xi's Methods of Treatment by Zhu Dan-xi, trans. by Yang Shou-zhong. ISBN 0-936185-50-3, $21.95

HOW TO WRITE A TCM HERBAL FORMULA A Logical Methodology for the Formulation & Administration of Chinese Herbal Medicine in Decoction, by Bob Flaws, ISBN 0-936185-49-X, $10.95

FULFILLING THE ESSENCE: A Handbook of Traditional & Contemporary Chinese Treatments for Female Infertility by Bob Flaws. ISBN 0-936185-48-1, $19.95

STATEMENTS OF FACT IN TRADITIONAL CHINESE MEDICINE by Bob Flaws. ISBN 0-936185-52-X, $10.95

IMPERIAL SECRETS OF HEALTH & LONGEVITY by Bob Flaws, ISBN 0-936185-51-1, $9.95

THE MEDICAL I CHING: Oracle of the Healer Within by Miki Shima, OMD, ISBN 0-936185-38-4, $19.95

THE SYSTEMATIC CLASSIC OF ACUPUNCTURE /MOXIBUSTION by Huang-fu Mi, trans. by Yang Shou-zhong and Charles Chace, ISBN 0-936185-29-5, hardback edition, $79.95

CHINESE PEDIATRIC MASSAGE THERAPY A Parent's & Practitioner's Guide to the Treatment and Prevention of Childhood Disease, by Fan Ya-li. ISBN 0-936185-54-6, $12.95

RECENT TCM RESEARCH FROM CHINA trans. by Bob Flaws & Charles Chace. ISBN 0-936185-56-2, $18.95PMS: Its Cause, Diagnosis & Treatment According to Traditional Chinese Medicine by Bob Flaws ISBN 0-936185-22-8 $18.95

EXTRA TREATISES BASED ON INVESTIGATION & INQUIRY: A Translation of Zhu Dan-xi's *Ge Zhi Yu Lun*, trans. by Yang Shou-zhong & Duan Wu-jin, ISBN 0-936185-53-8, $15.95

SOMETHING OLD, SOMETHING NEW; Essays on the TCM Description of Western Herbs,

THE DAO OF INCREASING LONGEVITY AND CONSERVING ONE'S LIFE by Anna Lin & Bob Flaws, ISBN 0-936185-24-4 $16.95

FIRE IN THE VALLEY: The TCM Diagnosis and Treatment of Vaginal Diseases by Bob Flaws ISBN 0-936185-25-2 $16.95

HIGHLIGHTS OF ANCIENT ACUPUNCTURE PRESCRIPTIONS trans. by Honora Lee Wolfe & Rose Crescenz ISBN 0-936185-23-6 $14.95

ARISAL OF THE CLEAR: A Simple Guide to Healthy Eating According to Traditional Chinese Medicine by Bob Flaws, ISBN #-936185-27-9 $8.95

CERVICAL DYSPLASIA & PROSTATE CANCER: HPV, A Hidden Link? by Bob Flaws, ISBN 0-936185-19-8 $23.95

PEDIATRIC BRONCHITIS: ITS CAUSE, DIAGNOSIS & TREATMENT ACCORDING TO TRADITIONAL CHINESE MEDICINE trans. by Gao Yu-li and Bob Flaws, ISBN 0-936185-26-0 $15.95

AIDS & ITS TREATMENT ACCORDING TO TRADITIONAL CHINESE MEDICINE by Huang Bing-shan, trans. by Fu-Di & Bob Flaws, ISBN 0-936185-28-7 $24.95

ACUTE ABDOMINAL SYNDROMES: Their Diagnosis & Treatment by Combined Chinese-Western Medicine by Alon Marcus, ISBN 0-936185-31-7 $16.95

MY SISTER, THE MOON: The Diagnosis & Treatment of Menstrual Diseases by Traditional Chinese Medicine by Bob Flaws, ISBN 0-936185-34-1, $24.95

FU QING-ZHU'S GYNECOLOGY trans. by Yang Shou-zhong and Liu Da-wei, ISBN 0-936185-35-X, $21.95

FLESHING OUT THE BONES: The Importance of Case Histories in Chinese Medicine by Charles Chace. ISBN 0-936185-30-9, $18.95

CLASSICAL MOXIBUSTION SKILLS IN CONTEMPORARY CLINICAL PRACTICE by Sung Baek, ISBN 0-936185-16-3 $10.95

MASTER TONG'S ACUPUNCTURE: An Ancient Lineage for Modern Practice, trans. and commentary by Miriam Lee, OMD, ISBN 0-936185-37-6, $19.95

A HANDBOOK OF TCM
UROLOGY & MALE
SEXUAL DYSFUNCTION by
Anna Lin, OMD, ISBN 0-936185-
36-8, $16.95

Li Dong-yuan's **TREATISE
ON THE SPLEEN &
STOMACH**, A Translation of
the *Pi Wei Lun* by Yang Shou-
zhong & Li Jian-yong, ISBN 0-
936185-41-4, $21.95

**PATH OF PREGNANCY,
VOL. I,** Gestational Disorders
by Bob Flaws, ISBN 0-936185-39-
2, $16.95

**PATH OF PREGNANCY,
VOL. II, Postpartum Diseases**
by Bob Flaws, ISBN
0-936185-42-2, $18.95

**How to Have a HEALTHY
PREGNANCY, HEALTHY
BIRTH with Traditional Chinese
Medicine** by Honora Lee Wolfe,
ISBN 0-936185-40-6, $9.95

**MASTER HUA'S CLASSIC
OF THE CENTRAL
VISCERA** by Hua Tuo, translated
by Yang Shou-zhong, ISBN 0-
936185-43-0, $21.95